Unstoppable Mental Toughness

The 12 Steps To Developing Unstoppable
Mental Toughness In Young Athletes
and High-Performance Sportspeople

Peter Estrop

Published by
Inspired Publishing Books
Inspired Publishing Ltd
27 Old Gloucester Street
London
WC1N 3AX

inspired publishing

ISBN- 978-1-78555-054-6

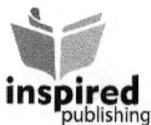

CONTENT

To my wife...without you, there would not be this book.

You are the one who believes in me all the time.

You are the one who inspired me.

You are everything to me.

Preface

It's often said that our lives are incredibly difficult in today's world. But actually, when you think about it, we are the billionaires of all of human history. This might sound contrary to what you believe, because we are constantly told that we live in the most dangerous, the most difficult, the hardest of times. News headlines tell us every day that crime is increasing, violence is rising, opportunities are fewer, jobs are scarce, and so on.

However, if you could lay out all of human history on a timeline, we are undoubtedly the richest, the most comfortable, the healthiest humans ever. As humans, we have never lived in such peaceful times before. And yet we are still crying, we are still miserable, we think we are so badly off. In comparison, the kings and queens of the past didn't live in the luxury that we do today. Think of it this way—even if you're on the poverty line, you are still far better off than at any other time in human history. Most of us at least have a warm bed, access to running water, and a toilet.

What we have today are incredible things available to us, but our minds are so soft that they only see what they don't have, rather than appreciating what they do have. People are so mentally weak these days that they can't even enjoy the greatest time in our history. But you do not have to be one of those people. You just need to develop mental toughness. Mental toughness is a huge factor in us appreciating what we have instead of seeing what we don't have.

Introduction

In life, many of us recognise the importance of developing mental toughness. We realise that it is a critical factor in unlocking our potential as individuals, and in becoming much more efficient and happy in our lives. People often wonder how it would feel if they could lock into their optimal mental state and perform at their best far more consistently. They know that it could be easier to achieve their goals and stay in a positive mental frame of mind. But most people don't know how to unlock this mental state and develop unstoppable mental toughness that will enable them to achieve their goals.

So, this book is for athletes, coaches, chief executives, managers, teenagers/young adults, those suffering with confidence problems, and many other people lacking in mental toughness. It's also ideal for those experiencing a mid-life crisis or burnout, and any individuals who want to finally achieve their goals. In every walk of life, **mental toughness is the key to success**.

We might not realise it, but the human mind offers multiple resources that can help us maximise our performance. We can develop the mental skills of grit, passion, perseverance, courage, determination, commitment, trust, and belief. Together, these skills make up mental toughness. They are the tools in the toolbox of mental toughness, and they can help us succeed. And when we develop these skills in mental toughness, it inevitably leads us to an even greater enjoyment of life.

Mental toughness is a rare commodity, but it can be a learned skill. In this book, you will develop the skills required for mental toughness. The examples included are predominantly from popular sports worldwide in order to illustrate the psychological principles of mental toughness. However, the examples are transferrable to all areas of life; these days, sports techniques are often applied in the business world and other performing environments. So, whether you're an athlete or a CEO, a teenager or a coach, the examples in this book can be applied to your home and working life. The skills required in mental toughness apply to any avenue of life.

In this book, I take a broad look at what mental toughness means in sport, business, and for individuals. I offer my definition of the concept based on my life experiences inside and outside of basketball, and the influences and lessons from my parents, coaches, teachers, teammates, friends, mentors, and colleagues over the years. I have had great fortune to witness real mental toughness in some amazing people I have met and situations I have been in. So, I relate examples and lessons of hard-won toughness I have seen up close, and that have had a positive and permanent impact on me. I would like to offer you these stories from my life, so you can look further into your own stories. Look into your past, pay attention to your present, and a create bright future.

Because I have lived with adversity for most of my life, I'm often asked: "How do you deal with this?" This book is my response to that question. *Mental toughness is the key to success.* Though my life experiences, I have discovered that all successful people share one trait—**psychological resistance**. The point is, I fail all the time, but it doesn't stop me from taking the next challenge. That mindset is critical for me in my career. And it will be critical for you too. You have to be willing to live with what you do, with the life you create for yourself, whatever the result. So never stop trying.

What you will get in this book

With many things in life, people want a recipe. With mental toughness, it is no different—people want a formula to build mental toughness. There are many recipes in this book, and I guarantee that if you follow the steps within them, you will get a favourable outcome.

This book will provide you with evidence of how important mental toughness is in our lives, show you why humans need mental toughness, and give you the knowledge you need to develop mental toughness. In this book, you will find out many things, including how to:

- Unlock your potential
- Build your confidence
- Improve your self-esteem
- Learn not to give up
- Achieve your best performance
- Become successful
- Be more effective
- Control your emotions
- Stay focused in any situation
- Overcome obstacles
- Be more self-disciplined
- Leave your comfort zone
- Cope with emotional stress and physical pain
- Be healthier
- Be happier
- Live longer
- Overcome burnout, a mid-life crisis, or bullying
- Develop positive behaviour
- Prepare yourself for real life
- Create a mindset of champions
- Increase your chances of finding the right partner
- Improve your diet
- Heal your pain
- Focus on the present and build a bright future
- Believe that anything is possible

- Start living your dream life

As a mental toughness expert, people often ask me how they can overcome a motivational slump, and focus better in critical situations. So, one of the primary aims of this book is to enable you to reproduce your optimal mental state and develop strategies that you can apply in real-world situations.

The information in this book will help you live a happier and healthier life, make your dreams a reality, and enable you to have a bigger impact, both in your life and in your work. In exchange for your promise to follow the steps, act on the information in this book, and commit to improving, I promise that I will provide you with information, ideas, and strategies that will help you develop mental toughness. Whatever strategies I suggest, whatever vision you have for your life, whatever goals you set for yourself can only become a reality if you have mental toughness.

How mental toughness works

Before we start, it's important that you understand how mental toughness works. It is basically like a muscle. To develop mental fortitude, just like if you want bigger biceps, you need to practice and work on it, so it can develop and grow. Although you're aiming to develop *mental* toughness, it is achieved through *practical*, physical action.

Every day, the choices you make will help develop your "mental toughness muscle". So you need to push yourself daily, even if it's only small steps at first. Mental toughness is developed through these **small wins**. And, if you can push yourself to make the small steps, you'll be able to keep walking when you face a challenge, and you'll be able to take the big leaps when you need to.

When things become challenging, most people give up and find something easier to do instead. But mentally tough people face a challenge, they see it as an opportunity, and they find a way to make it happen regardless. You will find a way to make it happen.

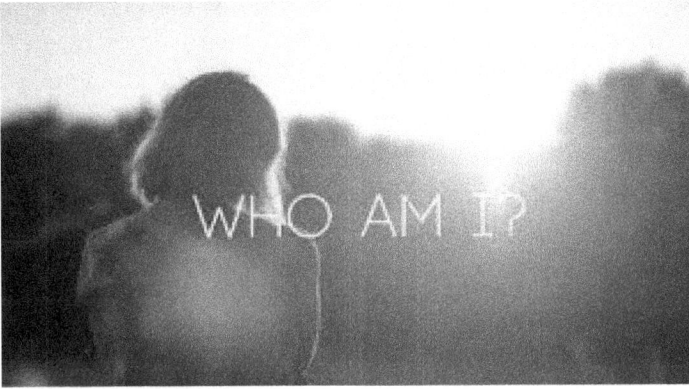

So, let me tell you a little about my background. I was born and raised in Gdansk, Poland, where on 1st September 1939, at 4.45 a.m., Poland was attacked. This attack is considered to be the beginning of the Second World War, which led to a loss of 70 million lives worldwide. The world would never be the same again, and it all started in my home town.

I was born as an only child during martial law in Poland. This was the period from 13th December 1981 to 22nd July 1983, when the authoritarian communist government of the People's Republic of Poland drastically restricted normal life by introducing martial law in an attempt to crush political opposition. Thousands of opposition activists went to jail without charge and as many as 91 were killed.

Martial law was lifted in 1983. During my early years, I experienced two systems: communism and young democracy. Communism was a time of tanks rolling along the streets most days, empty stores, propaganda, and censorship. The shortage of most essential products made everyday life a nightmare. During many of the various economic crises, store shelves were empty. Large shops supplied with only vinegar and Georgian tea are a commonly recalled flashback of the communist period. I often stood in a line for weeks with my mum to buy something (a book for example). There were periods when the availability of anything but basic goods was *none*. It was irritating.

Furthermore, most products were subject to a rationing system, which made some products available only to the bearers of unique cards. All of these nuisances resulted in what is known as a 'queue culture'. Families would queue for days to get a washing machine, a pram, or a pound of meat. Lines for everything, and poor-quality goods. Casual queueing investigators watched the order of the lines, and retirees would make additional money by being a 'stander' (known as a "stack" in Polish)—a person who stands in a queue for somebody else.

To have a phone line allocated and installed, someone could wait as long as 20 years. By comparison, in the Western world, it took one phone call and the next day you could have your landline installed. The deficit of personal phones was not only a result of poor infrastructure, but also because it was considered a very low priority by those in power. Fewer phones meant fewer conversations to control, less conspiracies, and little trouble.

The problem is that most people are not satisfied with a "cafeteria menu life" like this. Most people have the need or desire to do something unique, something that a uniformly planned society doesn't have on the menu. Somebody wants to see Greenland—sorry, no travel allowed. Someone wants to read an Argentinian poet—sorry, literature has to be read by a censor first, and that department is busy with other jobs. Someone wants to have a different colour in their room—sorry, you need to wait for the next 5-year plan for this colour to be available. Someone wants to do innovative cardiac surgery—sorry, our industry does not provide the surgical tools you need, and you are not allowed to (and you have no money to) buy them from somewhere else.

So, a curious mindset arose. People who would never have wanted to travel abroad if they had been allowed to started suffering from feelings like "I wouldn't be able to if I wanted to". The feeling of being restricted in everything became prevalent. Humans just work this way—put a person in a room that they may leave freely at any moment and they will most often stay there and make themselves busy with other things. But lock the door and the person will think of nothing other than getting out.

The second system, in my early days, was a young democracy, which started in 1989. Suddenly, almost overnight, there was a free market economy. Some people were shocked by the rise in unemployment and inequality. But then individuals were hired to do crazy things such as open doors in restaurants, develop new businesses, and so on. Suddenly, you could buy a washing machine just like that—in the shop—without queuing for three days! Nearly any product you wanted that had been impossible to purchase a few months ago, you could now get immediately. But to have a flat or a house now, you needed to get a mortgage from the bank and work hard to pay it off. In the old system, you could get an apartment for free (though sometimes you had to wait for 10 or 20 years for it if you didn't know someone in the government). Of course, not everybody was able to adapt to this entirely new system.

As a young boy, I had to adjust to this new reality. I was not born tough, but I saw toughness every day growing up. Every day, my parents got up and went to work. I learned about their work ethic, not from them talking about it, but from watching them do it. I'll never forget for how many years during the winter, I wanted to stay in bed and sleep all morning. I didn't want to get up early and go to school. But my mum never let me do this and always said "Get up now!" If I didn't get up on time, then my father used to open all the windows in my room and take the duvet off my bed! In the winter, it was often minus 25C. So after a few minutes, I always got up. It took me a while to understand why they never let me stay in bed and miss a day of school. The answer was, they didn't want me to be soft and have the option of giving up. This helped me to toughen up. Though in my early years, I didn't concentrate on toughness or even understand what it really meant.

The thing is, we are not born tough. We may be born into a great family situation or a difficult family situation that forces or conditions us to be tough, but we weren't born that way. Mental

13

toughness isn't a natural ability. You develop this toughness from experiences in your life—how you handle them, what you learn from them, and how you find your way through them guided by other people.

Mental toughness is more about having a "can do" attitude than about natural ability. The effort you put in is what creates success. Results are a measure of your current work, and failure is an opportunity to grow—not to give up. In a way, living in Poland helped me to better understand never to give up. If Polish people gave up during a tough time, Poland would not exist today. So today, I feel okay with failure as long as I know I have done everything I can to succeed.

What Is Mental Toughness? And Why Is Mental Toughness So Necessary?

Before you begin discovering how to develop mental toughness in the next chapter, it's important that you understand what mental toughness is, what it looks like in the real world, why it's vital, and when we need it. In particular, we'll look at the role of mental toughness for:

- Chief executives or managers
- Teenagers or young people
- Individuals at home or at work
- Sports people or athletes

What is mental toughness?

The first thing you need to realise is that mental toughness is about your **attitude**—it's not about your natural ability. It's about consistently doing something that you know you need to do to achieve your goals. It's about being committed to practicing daily, adhering to your programme or timeline, and not giving up. It's *not* about being naturally talented, innately intelligent, or physically strong.

14

You might doubt this, but I've seen it from personal experience. For two years, I studied management at the Compass Management Academy in the UK. At the start, they made us undertake psychological tests to see the limits of our individual mental and emotional capacities, as often happens at training academies. You'd probably expect that the people who made it through the Academy were those who had been determined as the "most intelligent", or had the most innate leadership skills.

But on the contrary, intelligence—and even leadership potential—weren't the key factors that influenced whether someone would graduate in Management. In fact, what made the difference was **perseverance** and having the **passion** to succeed.

You might think that these results were just a fluke or were limited to the Management Academy, but University of Pennsylvania researchers discovered the exact same when studying U.S. Army cadets trying to pass initiation. Rather than intelligence, physical strength, or size—the determining factor in their success was "grit". In case you're wondering, "grit" means having the passion and perseverance to achieve long-term goals, and it's measured on the "grit scale".

The researchers discovered that being just one standard deviation higher on the grit scale equated to a 60% likelihood of success—not good genes, not a high IQ, not innate talent (Duckworth et al., 2007). How does this link to mental toughness, you ask? Well, "grit" is basically a synonym of mental toughness, but I prefer the term "mental toughness" as it's easier to visualise and understand. But what does mental toughness, or "grit", actually comprise? In this book, we'll consider mental toughness as being comprised of:

Mental Toughness = Passion + Courage + Trust + Belief + Determination + Perseverance + Commitment

To develop mental toughness, you need the right mindset, and this involves personal self-awareness, self-confidence, and self-belief. You need to set goals for your life and be passionate about them.

You need the right skills and abilities: to be disciplined, able to concentrate, and able to say "no" so you can turn your goals into positive habits. You need the right approach: to be open to criticism, open to change, and committed to developing 24/7. You need to be able to navigate negative thinking, turn problems into opportunities, and win against adversity.

When is mental toughness important?

You've seen that mental toughness is a key factor in passing a management academy or cadet training, but how does this apply to other situations? In other words, if you're not training to become a manager or join the army, is "grit" or mental toughness still relevant? The answer is still a resounding **yes**.

Duckworth's research also demonstrated that mental toughness is a key component in all levels of education, from spelling bees at a young age through to graduates from Ivy League universities. The key factor in success for all of these was mental toughness—commitment to practicing and courage to keep going—rather than IQ or innate talent.

Moreover, she found that in the world of work, "grit" is the contributing factor in success and high performance. Duckworth and her researchers interviewed people working in fields that ranged from finance to the arts, medicine to government. The result was somewhat surprising, "Asked what quality distinguishes star performers in their respective fields, these individuals cited grit or a close synonym as often as talent" (Duckworth et al., 2007).

This demonstrates the importance of mental toughness not just in academia, but in any area of work, in any job you do, in any industry. It also follows through to every part of your life—including your health and wellbeing. In every situation, more than any other factor, what really makes a difference is your mental toughness: your commitment to succeed, your perseverance to make it happen, and your passion to achieve your goals. **Not your talent.**

You don't need to just take my word for it, or Duckworth's word. Think about it for yourself. Think back to all the times you saw a loved one waste their natural talent because they had no courage. Or an intelligent colleague fails to succeed because they lacked passion. Or your gym buddy gives up on getting bigger because they didn't persevere. We see these examples all the time in our day-to-day lives. If we're being honest, we have probably committed these sins ourselves at some point.

So, the answer to the question—*when is mental toughness is important?*—is **all the time, every day, in every situation**.

What does mental toughness actually look like?

So, now you know what mental toughness is and when it's required. But you might be wondering what it actually looks like in practice. Rather than an intangible concept on a page, how do you identify mental toughness in everyday life?

- In management, mental toughness is easy to spot in leaders and CEOs who display a clear vision for their company and strive to achieve it every single day. They don't get derailed by naysayers, finances, or a heavy workload.
- In sport, mental toughness is visible in those athletes who train hard every day, practice every day, and take responsibility for their own success. They don't give up despite injuries, setbacks, or rejection.
- In work, mental toughness is apparent in any worker who develops a habit of working hard every day to a plan, rather than haphazardly when they feel like it. They don't get side-tracked by demotivation, challenging tasks, or boring duties.
- On an individual, personal level, mental toughness is evident in those who put in effort every day to improve themselves to achieve their life's dreams. They don't get dissuaded by day-to-day life, lack of confidence, or limitations. And they certainly don't make excuses for not achieving what they want to.

- In teenagers and young people, mental toughness is seen in those who are developing the skills to succeed in the real world, as an adult. They set long-term goals for their life and are starting to make them happen in small ways every day. They are not preoccupied with playing video games, putting things off until they are an adult, or avoiding helping out at home.

Do you see one key similarity in each of these descriptions of real-life actions? The key word in each point is "**every day**". And by this, I don't mean just make an effort once every day and then forget about it for the rest of the day. What I mean is that you develop and display mental toughness through **consistent** effort, until it becomes a habit. As with most things in life, with mental toughness, consistency is key. So, don't worry if your life doesn't look like these descriptions right now, as mental toughness can be developed—and it will be in this book.

Next, we'll look more in-depth at mental toughness for each of these particular groups of people. Feel free to skip ahead to the section that is relevant to you.

What is mental toughness for managers, leaders, and chief executives?

If you are a leader, a manager, or a chief executive (CEO) and you want to become more efficient in your job and improve your leadership skills, then it's vital that you develop mental toughness in order to succeed. As you saw earlier, mental strength is more likely to determine your success than any other factor.

You might think I'm over-exaggerating here, but evidence shows that good leadership inherently relies on your mental strength. As a manager, mental toughness isn't about being able to charm people with fancy vocabulary or recite last quarter's sales figures from memory. It's not about your book smarts, or your IQ. It's also not about aiming for short-term gains.

For managers, mental toughness *is* about having **a mindset of champions**. This mindset enables you to pursue a long-term vision and overcome any challenges on the way. Champions don't aim to win a gold medal once and then throw in the towel. Champions wants to stay champions. So they set long-term goals. As a manager, you need to set the long-term vision for your company and anticipate the future, not just set short-term goals focused on the now.

What's more, you won't just accept that things are the way they are and think that there's nothing you can (or should) do about it. In the workplace, you often hear the phrase "But that's the way things have always been done" or "We don't do things like that around here". Mentally tough managers don't do things the way they've always been done—instead, they are **committed to continuous improvement**. Rather than resting on old laurels and traditional practices, they embrace progression. Mentally strong managers are always moving forward, never standing still.

In the workplace, you often hear the phrase "best practices" banded around. But best practices are static. They suggest that we should reach this "best" and then stop. Assume that the world around us isn't changing every day. Instead, I want you to banish "best practices" and adopt a new concept— "next practices". These practices are about continually improving, progressing, and transforming. They're about thinking "What's next?" and "How can we improve?"

Think about it—does a champion win the gold medal and then carry on training and working exactly as they did before? A champion realises their competitors are trying to take that gold medal, and they up the ante. They strive to improve so they can keep winning that gold. And they face every challenger with anticipation.

As a leader, you need to approach every challenge like the champion—with determination. Being a leader doesn't mean avoiding challenges or pretending they don't exist. In fact, leaders who are mentally tough embrace challenge because it helps them become better, faster, and smarter. As a mentally strong leader, you will face battles head on, and you won't give up when the going gets tough. You'll find a way to make it happen.

Step into the unknown, face your fears head on, put in all of your effort, and get back up when you're knocked down. The very foundation of mental toughness is having the courage to do these things. When you have this determination and this courage as a manager, you will be able to cope with a changing world and varying demands. You will be able to make it through any challenging situation with your team behind you.

A mentally tough leader needs to inspire their team to take action, show them the long-term vision, and bring them along on the journey. They need to turn failures into opportunities for learning and improving. In short, they need to encourage their employees to also develop mental toughness and a mindset of champions.

On a personal level, to do all of this, you must become a master of your emotions. As a mentally strong individual, you will be able to stay calm and know that you will make it through any difficult situation at work or at home. The great thing is that developing mental toughness as a manager has added extras.

Your journey of workplace growth will lead to improved self-esteem, knowledge, and personal growth. This means you will be able to deal with stress and other difficulties in your personal life, as well as those bigger strategic elements at work. This is vital, because your role as a high-level manager or CEO is likely to come with a lot of responsibility, and mental toughness will enable you to balance your work and home life. Mental toughness is as important and influential in your personal life as your work life.

So, mental toughness for leaders is:

- Having a mindset of champions
- Setting a long-term vision for success, not short-term gains
- Being committed to continuous improvement, not doing things the way they've always been done
- Striving for next practices, rather than best practices
- Facing challenges head on with determination and embracing challenges as a way to improve
- Encouraging your employees or team to also develop mental toughness

The great news is that you can easily develop mental toughness and this mindset of champions yourself with practice.

What is mental toughness for teenagers?

If you have children, you might be wondering how mental toughness can help them to succeed. Or, if you are a teenager or young adult who hasn't yet entered the working world, you may be unsure whether this book applies to you. The answer is that mental toughness will help everyone succeed. This section will cover mental toughness as a parent and as a teenager.

Parenting for Mental Toughness

As a parent, it's vital that you ensure your children develop mental toughness if you want them to grow up into capable, resilient adults who achieve great things and aren't a burden on society. Unfortunately, most parents don't realise the importance of their role in influencing who their children become as adults, or they take the wrong approach to parenting.

As a basketball coach, I've noticed that there tends to be two types of parents. The first kind are the majority, and their parenting style is too soft. The second kind are too hard. Over time, most parents have been raising children to be soft, weak, and ill-prepared for life in the real world outside of school or mum's apron strings.

Modern Parenting Doesn't Work

On the court, many parents try to protect their children from failing, from losing games, but this means their children grow up unable to deal with real life. Real life involves failure—we don't always win—and children need to learn this. If they grow up thinking they will always be the winner, they won't be able to cope with failure when it inevitably happens to them.

What's more, these parents seem to think they must do everything for their children while their children must do nothing, or do very little. They think that children should just enjoy their life, go to school, have fun with their friends, play games, and have no responsibilities—in other words, have an easy life. But this doesn't prepare them for *real* life, which isn't easy.

Instead, we raise children who believe their parents will do everything for them and give them everything they want, and when they become adults, they don't even know how to do basic things such as make the bed. It means parents having to arrange job interviews for their 18-year-old child or having children who never leave home. When your children grow up, they will have to leave home, get a job, pay their bills, and overcome difficult situations. Be honest with yourself, are you raising a child who is able to do these things? Or one who will struggle at the first hurdle?

With this soft parenting approach, we're creating a generation of young people who largely expect that things will just land in their laps, who are unable to overcome problems, and who aren't prepared for hard work or the real world. We're raising the next generation of adults to have little resilience. Added to this, the rise of the internet has led to a culture of cyberbullying, body shaming, and image consciousness.

It's no surprise then that depression, anxiety, and eating disorder rates among teenagers and young people have increased by 50-75% in the last 25 years. This might make you think you need to wrap your child up in cotton wool, to prevent them from ever being hurt, but on the contrary, the best thing you can do for them is help them develop the skills to survive their adult life.

I know it can be difficult when you feel that you don't have time to control your children and watch what they're doing all the time, when you're working what feels like 24/7 to pay for their lifestyle. You might think you're helping your child now by working all hours to give them everything they want, but in the long term, you're doing them no favours. You're turning them into someone who can't cope with the real world. Someone who will grow up unable to achieve things for themselves.

What many parents fail to realise or accept is that their children's behaviour is a result of their own behaviour, actions, and words. How you parent your children influences how your children behave and the adults they will grow up to be. So you need to take ownership of how you parent your children now if you want them to grow up to be strong, capable adults. You need to help them become mentally tough.

On the other hand, I also see parents who have unrealistic expectations of their children and who see "winning" as the most important thing. Helping your child become mentally tough isn't the same as being hard on them. These parents tell their children they must win every time, punish their children for losing, and express disappointment when their child makes a mistake.

Whether it's in sports or exams, taking this approach causes your child to be scared of failure, because your reaction comes across as disapproval or disappointment in them. They don't want to take part for themselves, or for enjoyment, but because they feel that winning is how they will get your approval and love. Children need to learn to cope with failure, not be scared of it and your reaction to it.

You need to accept that your child won't always win the race or the game. Your child should never feel they have to win or pass exams just to please you or be good enough for you. Instead of having a go at them for losing or making a mistake, help them to see how they can improve, help them take something useful from the experience and do better next time. Cheer your child on even if they make a mistake. Importantly, encourage your child to enjoy the experience. They will perform better when they enjoy it, particularly in sport, rather than when there is a heap of pressure on them from you.

Tell them you're proud of how much *effort* they put in—rather than being proud of them for simply being the winner. If you show your child that effort is just as important as coming first, they will develop the mental toughness to succeed and overcome hurdles in life. They need to see that "winning" isn't just about coming first, but about putting all of their effort in and being sportsmanlike. If they came first by pushing another child over, that's not winning. If they came second but put all of their effort in, don't berate them for not coming first.

Mentally tough parenting
As a parent, you can help your child develop the right mindset, skills, and approach to deal with life:

- Take care of your own mental health, as your children look after you and often model their behaviour on yours—be confident, think positively.
- Be the person you want your children to be.
- Accept your children for who they are, especially when they make mistakes or fail.
- Make your children help out at home rather than just playing games.
- Teach them the value of things rather than just buying them everything they want.
- Don't work all hours to provide them with a lifestyle—provide them with you as a parent.
- Don't expect them to win all of the time, and show them you're proud of their efforts.

- Show your child that winning is about trying their best, not about being the winner.
- Don't punish your child for making mistakes or failing.
- Teach them mental toughness by asking them what they learned from every experience, especially their failures and mistakes.
- Encourage your child to view each situation from different perspectives.
- Don't give your children advice, but ask them questions so they can discover the answers for themselves. If you do need to give advice, do it in a non-judgemental way.
- Communicate honestly and openly with your children.
- Explain the dangers of the internet, drugs, and alcohol. Keep an eye on them in these areas.

Mental Toughness For Teenagers

When you're a teenager or young adult, it can be easy to think that you're not good enough, you don't have enough natural talent, or you're not as good as others. I know because I felt like that myself. But I want you to forget that thought.

It doesn't matter whether you're a loud person or a quiet person, whether you're popular or not, whether you're "sporty" or "smart". It's not about your personality. It's not about how physically strong you are or naturally clever you are. You can succeed in life, in sport, in exams, and later in your jobs and relationships—in whatever you want to succeed in. You just need to be mentally tough.

To do this, you need to be able to control your emotions. When you're about to face a challenge, such as a high-pressure sports game or an exam, stay calm, take a deep breath, and focus on just that task. After the situation has ended, whether you won the game or not, think about what you learned from the experience, what you can do differently next time, what positive thing you discovered about yourself.

I know it can be difficult to see something good in yourself, but really think about it. Did you put in your best efforts? Did you surprise yourself? Did you pick up an opposition player when they fell down? Did you encourage your teammates to keep going when you conceded a point? Did you miss a goal but score the next one?

Don't worry about failing. If you're about to take an exam, you might be preoccupied with whether you pass it. But don't think about that now. The important thing is to focus on taking the exam and doing the best you can. Just think, even if you fail, you can improve in the future. You can always do better next time. It's more important that you put all of your effort in, rather than getting the highest marks.

If you do fail, use the experience as a learning opportunity. Think about how you can improve in the future and what you could do differently next time. If you fail an exam or lose a game, it can be easy to be hard on yourself. But it's important that you don't punish yourself for failing, or be mean to yourself. Remember that everyone fails from time to time. Don't tell yourself you're useless—say "I had a bad day but I can do better next time." Also, don't come up with excuses why you failed. Take responsibility for your performance, for your actions, and promise yourself you'll do better next time.

If you feel upset or angry, you can express this constructively through a creative channel, such as music, art, or even exercise. Stay calm, take a deep breath, and express your feelings in a healthy way. Don't give into the urge to be destructive or aggressive. If you're feeling like this, talk honestly with your parents or coaches. Tell them how you're feeling.

Sometimes, you might feel like you're competing against everyone else on your sports team, or in your class, but you need to realise that your only competitor is yourself. Stop comparing yourself to other people. Forget about beating other people, coming first, or getting the highest marks. Forget about winning. Just focus on being the best you can be, on improving yourself over time. You'll find that when you stop focusing on winning or losing, you'll feel more relaxed and will be able to concentrate on the race, game, or exam.

What is mental toughness for individuals at work and at home?

So, you understand the role of mental toughness if you're a manager, or when parenting your children, but what about you as an individual? What about at home and at work? The simple answer is that mental toughness is vital in **all areas of life**. It's the difference maker in parenting, work, sports, and home. It's what helps you people achieve your objectives in life while others fail.

The first, and most important, thing you need to understand is that success as an individual is not due to your innate talent or natural abilities. It's not about being "a natural with babies" or "made for the job". As you've seen, your ability and skills actually play a tiny role in your success—30% at the most. Instead, your success at work or at home is primarily down to your mental toughness. And this is great news, because you can't control your innate talent or your genetics, but you can develop mental toughness—and this means that **success is within your control**.

Whether you realise it or not, mental toughness is essential in all aspects of life. It's what helps you get through a bad break-up, a failed job interview, or a rough day. This is because mental toughness involves resilience, which is the capacity to recover quickly from bad experiences or difficulties. Whether we like it or not, failure is a natural part of human life, and we need to acknowledge this fact in order to develop mental toughness.

However, acknowledging failure doesn't mean focusing on our failures—on the contrary, if we focus on our failures, our current performance suffers. This is because you can't focus on success in the present if you're thinking about a mistake you made in the past, even if it was five minutes ago. What's more, focusing on your failures can cause you to lose control of your emotions—creating anger or upset—and make you lose confidence in yourself. This all leads to an increased likelihood of further failure, creating a vicious circle effect.

Mental toughness means *realising* that failure happens, and when it does happen, staying in the moment, remaining calm and focused, and staying confident. To do this, you need to move on from your mistakes. Accept your error and focus on the present. If you do this, you can succeed through adversity. You can overcome any challenge and leap any obstacle at work or at home.

What is mental toughness for sports people?

Of all the groups of people I've just discussed, it's probably easiest to understand the role of mental toughness for sportspeople and athletes. This is because sportspeople are always competing, always faced with challenges, and always aiming to win. Even from a young age, taking part in sports has a highly competitive element. While we might experience excitement, fun, and camaraderie, what drives us in both team and individual sports is the desire to win. We want to be the best. The strongest. The fastest. The most powerful.

Many sports psychologists and professionals have considered what makes someone the winner and the other the loser. This includes lecturer Dr Michael Sheard in his book *The Achievement Mindset: Understanding Mental Toughness (2008)*. Sheard questions why some sportspeople overcome adversity while others fail to, why some athletes go on to win the game even after committing a major error, and why some players allow difficulties during the game to affect them. He quickly discovered the reason for these differences. You guessed it—it's not technique, innate talent, physical prowess, or natural sporting ability—but mental toughness. When athletes develop mental toughness, and all of its component parts, they can overcome these adverse situations and go on to win.

Just a few years ago, mental toughness was a rarely explored and even more rarely understood area. It wasn't something that coaches or scouts sought in players, rather looking for raw talent. But now, the undeniable effect of mental toughness in sports has created a huge surge in interest in the field from players, coaches, managers, sports psychologists, and owners of sports teams. As a result, they're now looking for mental toughness in players.

The reason why mental toughness is so significant for sportspeople is because they spend their daily lives facing challenges, either to beat an opponent or to beat their previous best. When we face any difficulty, whether we succeed or not depends on our ability to manage both the internal and external demands on us. This means dealing with our physical environment and capability to overcome it, and our internal environment, that is, our mind—our thoughts, emotions, and beliefs.

The trouble is, many sportspeople focus primarily on the external— their physical ability, innate talent, and natural skills—while they neglect the internal aspects. But to truly succeed, they need to take a step further and look inside themselves. They need to optimise their minds, not just their bodies. Sportspeople work unceasingly to develop their muscles, but don't realise that the brain also behaves like a muscle. And it too needs to be developed. That's why athletes who work on their mental state achieve success much more than whose who don't.

While innate skill, ability, or talent accounts for up to 30% of our achievement, a staggering 60% is down to our attitude, our resilience, and our mental toughness. Researchers have even stated that as much as 85-90% of competitive sports are actually a mental game (Bhambri et al., 2005). This sounds crazy, but it makes sense when you consider that our brain is the control centre of our body. Our brain is what sends signals for our muscles to move, for us to make an action, and for us to keep going. It doesn't matter how much power is in your legs if your brain doesn't tell them to keep running.

In short, a sportsperson must have complete control over their mind as well as their body. If they neglect their mind, their body will be less capable of achieving success alone. Always remember that our minds and our bodies are inherently linked. What we think affects how we perform. If we think we're going to be terrible at something, we will be exactly that. Our confidence in our ability to achieve something actually helps us achieve it.

This is why you often see sportspeople who achieve great success even though they don't "fit the mould", that is, they don't look like what people expect of a sports star. Perhaps they're not very tall, don't look that strong, or have a disability, and yet they surprise us all by surpassing their competitors. It's because these players have mental strength, while their rivals don't. Despite their natural physical deficiency in comparison to their rivals, the mentally tough player is often the one who wins.

It's also why you find players who seem to have the physique needed to win, yet somehow never do. Or who have the talent and yet burn out, rather than experiencing a long-term sports career. Or who squander their natural ability. This is because natural talent doesn't automatically mean "winner"—if it did, we'd just hand the medals out without even competing.

Yes, you heard me right. What makes the difference between a winner and a loser is **mental toughness**: mental preparation and mental strength, especially when all other factors are equal. If your physical skills and abilities are the same as your competitors, developing mental toughness gives you the edge.

And it's not just in competitions that mental toughness makes a difference. In any sport, athletes often face high-pressure situations, but particularly in elite sports, these situations are known to be incredibly stressful and psychologically taxing. Developing mental toughness enables athletes to focus and control their minds in even the most stressful of environments, the most high pressure of situations—be it a gold medal race, a title bout, or in front of their first big crowd.

Whether you are naturally talented or not, you can boost your success by developing mental toughness and training your brain as well as your body. You need to develop optimum mental health, not just physical health. So, if you're a coach, you need to encourage your players to develop mental strength, and if you're an athlete, you need to train mentally as well as physically.

Hear it from the experts

I'm sure you don't need much more convincing, but in case you do, I can tell you that former NFL star and former head coach of the New York Jets Herm Edwards agrees that real toughness is completely mental. "The brain is a powerful thing," he said. "When you can weaken a man's mind, you've got him. When you can take a man's will away, take him beyond the limit of his toughness, you've got him."

Unfortunately, when things get tough, in sports and in life, too many people give up the fight. Edwards believes this taking the easy way out. He has always said, "You finish, or you retire". Truly tough people don't quit and they don't give in. The good thing is— Edwards also believes that kind of toughness can be taught, and that players actually welcome it.

Similarly, Super Bowl-winning NFL coach Jon Gruden of the Tampa Bay Buccaneers also believes that toughness can be taught, and if a leader sets a strong precedent, people will rise to meet a higher standard of toughness, so he always showed toughness to his teams and players. He said, "You have to coach toughness, the effort and discipline it takes to be excellent, every bit as much, if not more so, than Xs and Os or strategy." Gruden acknowledges that having the right mindset and mental conditioning can make anyone tougher than when they started. And that attitude won him a Super Bowl.

You often hear the word "talent" in the sports industry, and some players believe they don't have to work hard because they're "talented". They think it's okay to skip practise to hang out with their friends. But talent doesn't build a long-term career or guarantee success. Everyone has some talent, but not all of us in life are successful, so talent alone isn't enough. NBA Champion and one of the greatest basketball players Dwayne Wade said, "All the new players who come into the NBA have got talent, but how far they get individually is based on how hard they train and how smart they take their steps".

How do I become more resilient?

When I tell people that mental toughness involves developing resilience, I always get asked the same question: *how can I become more resilient?* As much as we might wish it did, resilience doesn't come from taking the easy road in life. To develop resilience, you have to face challenges and adversity so you can overcome them the next time round. This is why people who talk about resilience use the phrase "what doesn't kill you makes you stronger".

In other words, any time you've experienced a rough day, a setback, a failure, or poor performance, but you've made it through, then recognise this, use it to build your self-confidence, and realise you can overcome any situation. Many sports psychologists have a simple trick for this—creating a "trigger". This can be an action or word that helps you hit "pause" and reset, refocus, and carry on.

For example, say my boss has just called me into her office and told me I got last month's figures wrong. Instead of getting upset, reliving my mistake over and over again, or going home in a bad mood, I make a purposeful effort to clear my mind, let go of my mistake, and move on. This can be something as simple as rearranging the items on my desk, or drinking a glass of water—but this trigger action tells my mind that we're moving on.

As you drink the water, or move the items, you let go of your negative thoughts, feelings, emotions, and beliefs. It might sound odd, and at first it will feel like nothing is happening, but over time, your mind will understand the trigger and react accordingly.

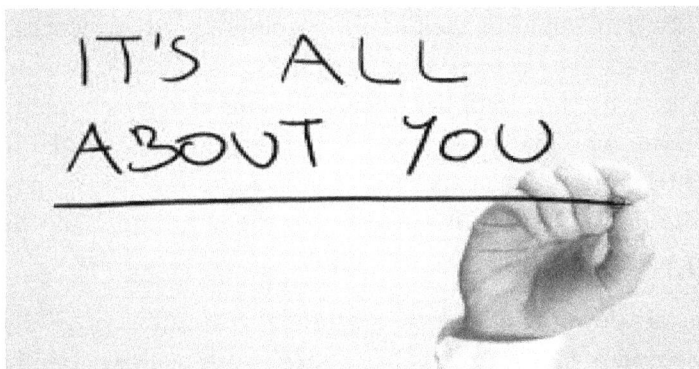

Simple Steps to Developing Unstoppable Mental Toughness in Everyday Life

How do you actually develop unstoppable mental toughness? Where do you start? In this chapter, we'll look at:

- How to start developing mental toughness in everyday life
- Six positive habits to get you started
- How mental toughness is about small wins

Where mental toughness is built

Firstly, let's clear up a misconception you might have. Although we've been talking about how mental toughness can help you succeed in big, high-pressure sporting events or business situations, mental toughness isn't just about how we react in these extraordinary circumstances. It's not just about how we were in the gold medal race, or how we fared in the Board meeting. Undoubtedly, these high-pressure situations test our mental toughness, but it's the everyday situations are where mental toughness is built.

Remember from the previous chapter that mental toughness is about everyday consistent effort? This means that **mental toughness is built on small wins**. Mentally strong people develop methods that support their daily success. In other words, they develop positive habits, and it's these habits that form the foundation of their rational beliefs and ultimately set them apart from those who don't succeed. They focus on the essential things, no matter how many challenges or difficulties life throws at them. And these habits make it possible for them to overcome the big challenges.

So to start developing mental toughness, you can begin with these six easy points that from my experience, work really well in the real world. While you do these things, always bear in mind that **mental toughness is about your habits, not about your motivation.** We all suffer from demotivation and lack of will power from time to time, but mental toughness involves developing habits that enable us to succeed regardless of how motivated we are.

1. Get straight up!

Although it's tempting to lie in bed and press snooze for 5 more minutes, or half an hour longer, develop the habit of getting up when your alarm goes off. Start your day as you mean to go on. After all, if you can't make yourself get out of bed in the morning, how can you achieve anything bigger than that? Yes, it feels nice to go back to sleep, but instead of giving into these feelings, acknowledge them, accept that you're still tired, and then get out of the damn bed.

2. Make your bed

As soon as you're out of bed, make the bed. It sounds like a tiny thing, but it's a small win. You're starting your day with a win. And you're developing discipline and organisation in the process. Mental toughness is about creating small daily rules, sticking to an agenda, and overcoming any difficulties over and over again, and making your bed is the first step on this path. It may make you smile, but this simple act is setting you up for success.

3. Do some exercise

The next step is doing something physical. The last thing you want to do in the morning is exercise, when you feel like you don't want to do anything, you're tired, you're not even properly awake yet, but just get into the habit of doing some exercise. Do something simple like push-ups by your bed, or go for a run, or to the gym. In the words of Drew Shamrock, "How many workouts have you missed because your mind, not your body, told you that you were tired?"

4. Plan your day

Every morning, write one, two, or three things that you **must** do today in your diary, phone, or on a piece of paper—particularly things that need to be done but that you don't really want to do. Then, when you get side-tracked throughout the day, look at your list and ask yourself, "Do I do the main tasks of the day, or do I waste my time?" When you realise you've got side-tracked, get back on track as quickly as possible and don't wallow in your failure to stay on track.

5. Do your homework first

When you get home from work or school, do your homework or jobs immediately. Don't put them off until later. It won't be fun, and you'd probably rather be putting your feet up or turning on the TV, but mental toughness is about doing things you don't want to do until you're comfortable doing them. It might be tough at first to make yourself do it, but when it becomes a habit, you won't even notice it.

6. Eat something you don't like

Every day, you should be eating healthily to keep your body in great condition. This can be difficult at first, especially if you prefer the taste of processed, sugary food, rather than healthy fruit and veg. So every day, switch something processed or unhealthy for something healthy that you don't like the taste of, and make yourself eat it. Most people learn to like the taste of new food after around 25 tastes, so doing this helps you to rise above your feelings and build mental toughness.

Small wins lead to big gains

These may sound like small things, but do not underestimate them, as they're incredibly powerful. If you do these six things consistently every day, you will develop the ability to rise above your feelings, and you will enable yourself to develop unstoppable mental toughness. Then, when something doesn't go your way in your day-to-day life, rising above your feelings will come easy to you, because you do it every day anyway. Remember, the important thing here is focusing on these small daily habits, not on trying to make life–changing transformations from day one.

You might be wondering why not just start with the big challenges, but the simple fact is, if you can't overcome the small daily challenges, how will you walk away as the victor from the real tough situations? When you can defeat these small challenges, you develop the mental strength to succeed in the toughest circumstances and the biggest challenges.

What's more, you can't develop mental strength if you don't challenge yourself every day. Remember, your brain is like a muscle, and when you challenge yourself every day in small ways, your mind grows and becomes more able to deal with challenges. Your mind increases in confidence, and next time you encounter the challenge, you know you can succeed because you've succeeded before.

In other words, you can't just *think yourself* to mental toughness. You can't imagine overcoming challenges, but never actually attempt them in the real world. **Mental strength is obtained through action, not thought.** Action is what tells your brain you can do it again next time. Action is what shows you that you can overcome challenges. So, don't just sit there thinking about it—actually do it!

Reminder

So, what does it look like when you encompass mental toughness?

- You never give up.
- You are resilient.
- You embrace the possibilities, not the problems.
- You recognise that everyone is facing a difficult battle.
- You keep trying to make a difference one person, one task, or one choice at a time.
- You understand that life is a marathon of making consistently good decisions every day.
- You look for the lessons and learn from your mistakes, but aren't paralysed by them.

In short, you decide to approach all of life's adventures, both good and bad, and move forward from each experience to consciously live your life with focus.

Mental toughness is an attitude of being committed to consistent daily action to improve ourselves and achieve our goals. To, to start developing mental strength:

- Rise above your feelings of not wanting to do something
- Challenge yourself daily through physical action
- Be consistent in your actions and efforts every day
- Develop positive habits
- Help yourself achieve small wins

In the following chapters, I'm going to show you a method to develop unstoppable mental toughness.

CHAPTER 1

Develop Self-Awareness

"Life isn't about finding yourself. Life is about creating yourself." George
Bernard Shaw

The first step in any process, on any journey in life, is always
critical—as it allows you to start your journey. Whatever your
destination, you must take the first step to get there. And to do this,
you have to understand that you are in charge of your life. You are
responsible for yourself. You make the decisions and you make a
choice—you, and no one else. It is not your friend, your neighbour,
your parent, or your grandmother telling you what your journey is; it
is always you. So you need to take control of your life. Every good
ship has a captain, and you are the captain of your life.

Self-awareness is the first step in developing mental toughness. This
is because in order to improve yourself, you need to have a realistic
view of yourself, including your strengths and your weaknesses.
When you have good self-awareness, you are able to make changes
to yourself and your life.

Take control

If you doubt this, if you think your life is not in your control, just
imagine this. You are holding your whole life in your hands like a
physical object and you give it to your friend saying, "Listen, this is

my life, and I'm giving it to you to make me famous and rich, get me a nice car and a lovely house, etc. I'm going to go back home and lie on the bed. Just let me know when that happens. Remember, don't let me down otherwise I'll not talk to you." This metaphor represents how we often blame others for our failure.

When you stop complaining and search for your solutions to the obstacles that life throws at you, you will realise that you are in charge of your journey and almost entirely in control of your life.

When you moan, you create bad habits and blame everything or everyone around you. So, when you grumble, you are going to fail! It is that simple! If you don't overcome this attitude, then no one else will do it for you. An individual who wants to be successful will find a way when a person who doesn't want to be successful will find excuses. So, take control of your life right now. Stop making excuses. And realise that only you can determine what happens in your life.

Develop self-awareness

Self Awareness & How to Develop it

Once you've taken control of your life, the next step is developing self-awareness. People often talk about self-awareness, but do we really practice it? We need to start, because it's a powerful tool to help us understand ourselves and why we behave the way we do. We can understand many of the difficulties we experience in life— from work to relationships, fears to stress—when we have self- awareness. It can help us improve our health, happiness, self- esteem, emotions, and behaviour. So, if self-awareness is so important for us, how can we achieve it?

Firstly, you need to understand that the majority of our actions are based on unconscious beliefs, desires, thoughts, or patterns. If we're not aware of why we're doing things, we can't make changes to them, even if we're aware that we are causing ourselves difficulties, that the path we're on isn't good for us. We're just acting, reacting, and behaving—without direction or thought. For example, I tell my friends that I want a promotion at work, and yet my actions are turning up late every day and failing to deliver my work on time. My actions tell me that subconsciously something is going wrong, because my actions don't match what I'm saying. Until I discover why I'm sabotaging myself, I won't get that promotion.

This is why self-awareness is vital. Self-awareness shines a light on the lies we tell ourselves and the false beliefs we punish ourselves with. By being aware of my unconscious thoughts, I might discover that I've been lying to myself and I'm actually incompetent at work—I want to be promoted because I'm not coping in my current role. Then I can do something about fixing it. Or maybe I believe that I don't deserve the promotion because I'm actually lacking self-confidence. When I figure out the reason, I can address the problem and start changing my actions.

The great thing is that you can develop self-awareness. Personally, I encourage self-awareness by spending 15 minutes meditating before I go to sleep every night. This doesn't mean surrounding myself with candles (though you can do that if you want!), but thinking back through my day and assessing where I made mistakes. If you don't want to meditate, you could write it down in a notepad, talk out loud to yourself, or talk to an honest loved one. The important thing is to engage in this self-reflection and be honest with your answers—don't let your mind trick you.

So, I ask myself the following questions:

- Did I get up when my alarm went off? Did I make my bed?
- Did I do some exercise?
- Did I eat healthily? Did I eat something I don't like?
- Did I do what I needed to today?
- Did I achieve the things on my to-do list?
- What did I learn today that was new?
- Was I kind and loving to others and to myself?
- Did I check social media 20 times today at work/school? Did it help me to complete my daily plan?
- Did I listen when people were talking to me?

If you do this simple, honest Q&A session with yourself at the end of each day, you'll wake up the next day with a better understanding of yourself, knowing how you need to improve and the pitfalls you need to avoid.

Self-awareness after failure

A great time for this reflection and self-awareness is after an argument, a setback, or a failure, which also helps you stop reacting emotionally to the event. When you fail, think about the event rationally and objectively, break it down into each part, and consider what went awry. Try to understand what really happened. Where were the errors? Were you missing some information?

When something goes wrong, we tend to feel unconfident and uncertain, so we sometimes react with anger, upset, or excuses. We also often misunderstand what actually happened. So if you're being consciously and actively aware, you're much more likely to solve the problem than if you're whinging to your friends about how unfair it is, or shouting at someone else about it in an attempt to shift the blame.

For example, if you've spent all day chatting to your friend on WhatsApp and you miss an important deadline, do you learn from your error and get back to work as quick as you can, or do you blame your friend for distracting you? Being self-aware means you need to be able to face yourself honestly. Instead of getting angry or upset, or making excuses, you need to quickly accept your mistakes, learn from the experience, and turn your awareness into positive action.

To be clear, admitting your errors and reflecting on what went wrong doesn't mean beating yourself up or wallowing in your mistakes. Self-awareness means taking responsibility for your life, your mistakes, and your actions—not overly berating yourself for getting things wrong. So, when you're analysing where things went wrong and owning your mistakes, have a little compassion for yourself. Developing self-awareness doesn't happen overnight—it will take time for your new positive habits to take hold, and your old negative beliefs to be overridden.

Finally, don't get discouraged if your journey of self-awareness becomes harder and harder. As you try to override your old beliefs with new ones, your mind will fight back and try to maintain the status quo. This is because it's easier to stay on the well-worn path we've been treading, as miserable and boggy as that path is, rather than finding a new, unknown path. Don't give in. Remember that mental toughness is about never giving in. **Tip**: When times get tough, it's great to remember an inspirational quote that gets you back on track. My favourite is "The harder you fall, the higher you can bounce back up."

Growing self-awareness

Self-awareness enables you to create a mind map of your unconscious habits, beliefs, thoughts, and desires. It helps us understand our minds. This mind map stops you falling back into old habits and repeating the same mistakes over and over again, like knowing which roads to avoid because there's always traffic or roadworks. This is just like when we use a spreadsheet at work to keep control of a budget, or maintain a food diary to ensure we're eating well. Without making the effort to create the spreadsheet or write the journal, we often lose track and overspend or forget what we're eating.

Self-awareness is like a muscle that grows over time, and ultimately gives us the strength to take action. Being self-aware means we are always consciously acting, instead of passively accepting our situation or reacting based on our subconscious thoughts. When we're self-aware, we cut out negative influences and replace them with positive habits. We become aware of our impulses, thoughts, and actions, and we enable ourselves to become our best selves.

Eventually, your purposeful and active efforts to be self-aware will lead to a strong sense of self-knowledge and self-confidence. You will know exactly who you are, why you react the way you do, and why you behave the way you do. In your awoken state of consciousness, you'll see the right path more clearly to achieve your goals. Decision-making will become easier, because you'll know exactly what you want. And your consciousness will extend to seeing the truth behind the behaviour of others. When all your actions integrate into your personality, you have achieved a state of being comfortable in your skin.

Self-awareness in leadership

If you're a manager or CEO, then self-awareness is vital to your success. This is because you are responsible for your organisation (or a part of an organisation), and the company is constantly affected by the environment it is in. Your business is likely to face changing circumstances, be it industry-related, legal obligations, or variations in demand. So as a leader, you need to be able to quickly adapt to these changes.

The first step in adapting to this change is understanding your own feelings, how your emotions affect your behaviour, and how your actions can affect the outcome. If you're not self-aware, then how can you modify your behaviour and actions accordingly to ensure your business weathers the storm? You'll simply be leaving the fate of your business up to chance, or you'll make an excuse that the result was out of your control.

For example, say your business needs to produce 25% extra this quarter to survive, but your employees are refusing to step up the pace. If you're aware of your own actions and behaviour, you might realise you are being ruled by your emotions. You're panicking that you won't meet the order and you're angry that your employees won't speed up. So, your actions are shouting at them and suggesting they are not being productive. Instead, you can modify your behaviour by explaining the situation, and ask them for their help to meet the order. This way, your self-awareness turns the situation in your favour, and you convince your employees to fight the battle with you.

Being aware of and managing your emotions is vital as a CEO or senior manager. If you can't see the effect that your feelings and behaviour have on your employees, then you need to spend some time thinking about this, or your employees will not react the way you want them to.

You might think that your business has been doing well enough without you being self-aware, but a lack of self-awareness only leads to short-term success. Eventually, your unaware actions will undermine the long-term achievement you are trying to build for yourself and your organisation.

Like other leadership skills, you can develop self-awareness—it just takes consistent effort. Be aware, developing self-awareness means you are likely to identify actions and behaviours that are damaging your company's success, so in the short term, it may need lead to upheaval. However, in the long term, self-awareness will enable your business to reach new heights of success.

Reminder

To start developing mental toughness within yourself, you need to:

- Take control of your life
- Stop making excuses
- Stop moaning and blaming others
- Develop self-awareness
- Do a Q&A session with yourself everyday—be honest with yourself
- Start with the six small daily habits

CHAPTER 2

Set Your Goals

"Start by doing what's necessary; then do what's possible, and suddenly you are doing the impossible" - Francis of Assisi

Setting goals is the second step in developing mental toughness. This is because to improve in any area, including yourself and your life, you need clear goals. You can't develop mental toughness without having goals to work towards or you'd just be wandering aimlessly or coasting through life.

What's more, goal setting doesn't just mean creating a life plan and being responsible for it, but about gaining the inspiration to aim high, dream big, and reach things that we thought were impossible for us. Setting goals gives you a powerful way to motivate yourself when you're developing mental toughness.

All of us would like to achieve something, be it big or small—but we don't always turn these "would likes" into clear, specific goals. So, in this chapter, you'll discover:

- Where to begin start with setting goals and finding your goal
- What happens when you don't set goals
- How to actually set clear goals
- Turning goals into actions

Set your starting point - A

Often, we don't realise how important is to consider our starting point. This is a fundamental mistake. You need to identify your starting point so you know where you're coming from. If you're not sure, your point of departure is **here and now**. Whatever part of life you need to work on, consider what position you are in right now—whether it's at home, in a relationship, at the gym, on the sports field, at work, or as a manager. How do you feel mentally and physically? What is your relationship with your employee, coach, friends, or partner? What is your position on the court, field, at work, or at school? How fast are you, how efficient, or how high can you jump?

I recommend that you write all of this down on a piece of paper and keep it in a safe place. It is crucial that you do this to find out exactly where you are on your journey map. We are only human, and we may not know or be able to see whether we are making progress on our journey or not. That's why you need a starting point. When you have a starting point, you can compare where you were when you started to where you are now. Every month, you can analyse where you are and see how far you have come.

Knowing your location on your journey map allows you to get to your destination quicker, because you're not wandering around aimlessly. It also enables you to see yourself in the bigger picture and be motivated by seeing your progress.

Know your finish line - Z

Now we've got our starting point, we need to know where our finish line is. This is all straightforward and logical. Your goal is like a compass that can show you which direction to go in. Without a clear goal, it's like playing a game of basketball without knowing where the basket is. You'll waste time and energy without a clear target. When you have a target, you will work to achieve it. If you want to improve in your chosen sport, then every day, every workout and training session is getting you a step closer to your dream—this is what happens between A and Z.

For example, I was training at a basketball team (South West U-16) and before the season, I set a goal for our team to rank in the top three for at least one of the top three international tournaments. We played in heavily-manned tournaments in the Czech Republic, Poland, and Belgium. The goal I made was clear to the team, and I wanted us to achieve it in the next six months. Every day, I imagined that we would succeed. We worked very hard, and our goal mobilised us in hard times. We managed to reach our aim and we entered the final in the tournament in Poland, where we won a silver medal.

Maybe you're reading this book and you're shy or you're afraid of dreaming. When you're setting your goals, don't be scared to dream, don't be afraid to set a goal that most people wouldn't even consider. Be brave enough to believe in your dreams. You are the one who can make your dreams happen. Sometimes, the greatest danger for us is not that our goal or aim is too high, but that it is too low and too easy for us to reach it.

If you're scared, you need to realise that everything you can imagine in your head is exactly what you can achieve. That's a fact. If you doubt this, consider the first flight to the moon, building the Empire State Building in New York and the Golden Gate Bridge in San Francisco, or creating Real Madrid—the most successful football team of all time. All of this was envisioned, pictured in someone's head first.

So, follow the example set by people who reached their dreamed destination or achieved success. All of those people who completed their journey had an "A to Z". They had a starting point and a target, and they did the hard work of getting from one to the other.

What happens when you don't set goals?

You've seen that goal setting is vital to achieve long-term success, so you might be wondering, why doesn't everyone do it? If it's so great, why isn't everyone jumping on the goals bandwagon? Well, there are a few very simple reasons, some of which you may have experienced yourself...

- **Fear of failure**—We are afraid of situations where we won't succeed, so we don't put ourselves out there and risk the pain of failing.
- **Fear of ridicule**—We worry about being ridiculed or rejected by others because our dreams seem silly or unachievable to them.
- **Fear of missing out on something else**—Sometimes, we think that by pursuing one thing, we're potentially missing out on other things.
- **Lack of knowledge**—Goal setting is not taught at school (although this should be compulsory in my opinion). This means many people have no idea why or how they should set goals.
- **Fear of success**—Sometimes, we are even scared of succeeding because it will lead to change.

Fear of failure

Often, the main reason we don't set goals is because we're scared of failing to achieve them. If this is the case, I want you to remember a famous line said by Teddy Roosevelt: "In any moment of decision, the best thing you can do is the right thing, the next best thing is the wrong thing, **and the worst thing you can do is nothing."**

In other words, doing nothing towards your dreams is worse than doing something and getting it wrong. Think of it this way, if you don't set a destination because you're scared of not reaching it, you'll coast through the sea of your life without steering your own ship, being blown wherever the wind takes you or wherever the strongest force pushes you. This isn't being the captain of your own life—it's being a passenger on someone else's journey. If you're following someone else's journey, then you're failing at your own.

Think about it—in the main areas of your life, are you following your own path, someone else's, or none at all? If you're being honest with yourself, the majority of your efforts are most likely spent on someone else's dreams. Whether it's working tirelessly to achieve the vision of your boss, playing in a position you don't want to play in, or doing the job your parents imagined for you. It's time to change that. If you're focusing on failure—remember, failure is a natural part of life. On your goal setting journey, you will inevitably fail at some point, but you can always get back up.

Fear of missing out on something else

How many times have you heard someone say they're "keeping their options open"? Whether it's in work, in relationships, or opening a new business, what this actually translates to is *doing nothing*. If you're keeping your options open because you're not sure where you want to go, you'll inevitably go nowhere. You'll miss out on everything in life.

If you spend your time worrying that by pursuing one path, you're missing out on another path, then you're already missing out. By doing this, you're not taking any path, and you're not going anywhere. Anything that happens in your life will be someone else's decision. You'll stay in a job you don't enjoy, stay with a partner who's not right for you, or miss out on a dream business opportunity. You'll accept other people's dreams as your own.

So, if you know you think this way, a well-known way to stop this at the end of every day is to put a big cross through that day in your calendar, or diary, and realise you're never getting that day back. Did you use it wisely? Did you miss out on anything? You'll quickly see that you're missing out anyway, that keeping your options open is really closing them off. So, choose a path, and keep going.

If you're scared of making the wrong choice, you probably don't know yourself well enough yet, and you need to develop more self-awareness. So, go back and learn about yourself, then come back to goal setting.

Fear of ridicule

When you're setting goals for yourself, you need to be aware that there will always be people who won't believe in what you want to achieve. They'll try to persuade you that you're not ready, you lack potential, or you're stupid. At every stage, there is someone who will ask you what on earth you're doing.

If someone tells you that you can't do this, then what they often mean is that they wouldn't be able to achieve it. Don't let anyone hold you back because of their insecurities. Be ready to face them. Prove people wrong. Demonstrate that you can achieve your goal. If you are true to yourself and that's not enough for the people around you, change the people around you!

When you take control of your life and decide the path you want to follow, you'll experience an overwhelming sense of power over your destiny. Don't be like everyone else simply wandering through their lives—take control and set the path for your dreams.

Lack of knowledge

When we're kids, we get asked all the time what we want to be when we grow up. Many of us had a dream job—like being an astronaut or an actor. But then we go to school, college, and even university without being taught how to actually achieve our dream jobs, or in fact, discovering that we need to set long-term career goals for ourselves.

So then, we graduate and take any job to pay the bills and live in the real world, or we take the job our parents think we should take, or we accept the job we think we're qualified for—rather than reaching higher, or dreaming big. If you don't set long-term goals, then you'll meander through your working life taking what is offered and pursuing other people's visions and dreams instead of your own. You'll be working towards the vision of your boss, not own. You might even get offered promotion after promotion and earn more than you expected, and you might deceive yourself into thinking that the promotions are great for a while.

But at some point in your career, you'll most likely feel lost, unhappy, or unfulfilled. You'll feel that somewhere along the line, you forgot to do what you wanted to do, or you got washed along in somebody else's tide. Maybe you even recognise questioning why you're doing the job you're doing. You might have earned a degree in archaeology and imagined travelling the world, but now you're working a desk job in accounting and wondering what went wrong.

If you want to direct the course of your own life, then it's essential that you set long-term goals and objectives to build your career. If we know ourselves, and we set long-term career goals from a young age, then we can achieve our dream jobs and enjoy fulfilling careers pursuing our own passions, instead of someone else's. I used to tell my basketball players before games or tournaments "You cannot influence the direction of the wind, but you can always set sails accordingly".

Fear of success

This might sound strange, but some people actually fear achieving success. This can be because they are scared of what might change if they achieve success, such as losing friends, having a different lifestyle, or having more responsibility, and so on. For example, they may be afraid that if they achieve huge success and suddenly become very wealthy or famous, their friends will think they have changed as a person and won't want to hang out any more.

If you are afraid of success, you are stopping yourself from achieving your potential. But don't worry, because you can overcome this. The first thing you need to do is some self-reflection. Think about what it is deep down that's causing your fear of success. If you think your friends will ditch you, perhaps you're actually worried about your relationships and need to work on them. If you're worried you won't know how to manage new-found wealth, perhaps you need to improve your knowledge of finance and work on your self-confidence. If you're scared of change, remember that you will be able to adapt to your new circumstances.

How to set actually goals

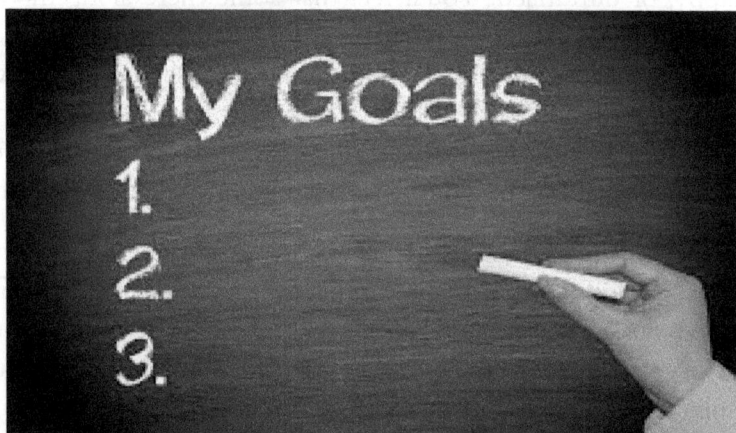

So, let's get down to actually setting some goals. You might have heard of the SMART method of goal setting. I personally find that setting SMART declarations is the best way to stay on course. A SMART goal is: **s**pecific, **m**easurable, **a**chievable, **r**ealistic, and **t**ime-related.

When you set goals, remember that you're setting a destination, not a direction. You might think you have a direction already, so you must have set some goals, right? This is just an illusion of movement. Consider this, the direction you're moving in is west, but your destination is a specific location—the sports field for example. Set your goals as **destinations, not directions**.

To start, ensure you write your goals down. There's no better way to lose track of your goals than by not writing them down. So, go and get a pen and paper right now. Write each letter of the SMART acronym down to ensure you're meeting each part of goal-setting.

Then, when you're writing your goals, ask yourself the question "Will I know when I've reached my destination?" This is because goals are answered with "yes" or "no". If I asked you "Have you reached your destination?", the answer can't be "possibly". You either have reached it or you haven't. To do this, you need to make your goals detailed—add dates, figures, times, locations, and amounts. These details ensure your goals are measurable, that you can easily check whether you've achieved them.

For example, if you set a vague goal of "lose weight", you might be uncertain whether you've achieved your goal and when you even need to check your progress. In contrast, a specific goal is "lose a stone in the next two months". After two months, it will be very clear whether you've achieved this goal or not.

Then, you need to turn your goals into positive affirmations of success. This means don't write goals that are negatives i.e. what you don't want. If you focus on what you don't want, that's exactly what you'll end up with it. So only write goals you *do* want. Similarly, avoid passive words like "might" or "probably", as they'll make your mind doubt that it can be achieved.

The next step is imagining you've already achieved them, and writing them down as if this is happening, for example, "This month, I am a stone lighter." Writing them in present tense builds your self-confidence that you can achieve them, like we looked at earlier.

If you find this task difficult, don't give up. Setting meaningful goals isn't easy, but it's worth it. It takes purposeful effort to set goals. But it's the only way to achieve success. If you're struggling to decide what you want, remember to be self-aware. When you know yourself completely, setting goals is much easier.

Goal setting as a sportsperson

When you play for a sports team, your coach or team manager may set a direction for you and help you to develop skills in a position that suits the club's need, but that doesn't necessary suit you or meet your goals. For example, they might need you to be a running back because they're lacking players in that position, while you have a goal to become the star quarterback. While it's good to help your team and develop new skills, you always need to have your own personal goals and work on improving the area of your game where your goals lie. This will help you to become a more complete player and a player with higher value.

Goal setting at work

So, if you've been getting up every morning and going to work at a job that isn't in line with your goals, take this time to set long-term career goals for yourself. Really think about what you want to achieve in life, and then write a specific, detailed description of where you want to be this time next year in terms of SMART goals. For example, I was working in a job that wasn't in line with my goals, and I wanted to be a basketball coach, so while I was on the bus to work, I used to write this detailed plan that would enable me to become a basketball coach.

Goal setting as a CEO

If you're a CEO of a business, you probably think "I'm already following my own goals." After all, you set the direction of the company and possibly even created it, right? But when you think about it, are you *really* following your own goals? Or are you following the goals set by your shareholders, other stakeholders, the local council, the public, or your partners—and trying to convince yourself that these are your goals?

You might think goals like "increase the company's profits" or "expand into other markets" are fine, but they're too vague. You need to be more specific in your goals such as "Open a new business in five new countries across the world that are turning a 10% profit within the next 18 months". Then your affirmation would be "This year, I am turning a 10% profit in five new global businesses."

Then ensure that your goals as a CEO align with your goals as an individual and that you haven't lost track of your personal goals. To be successful as a CEO, you need to be happy as an individual too. You need to ask yourself what your personal goals are? Where would you like to be in a few years? Are you happy at the moment? Do your personal goals match your business goals?

Finally, your employees need to understand the company strategy in order to help you fulfil your goals. In a high-stress position such as CEO, it's easy to lose track of your goals, so it's helpful to do regular reviews. The Pareto 80/20 rule works well as a CEO, so 80% of your goals may be personal and 20% to fulfil the goals of your shareholders or stakeholders.

Turn goals into actions

Great, you've set some goals. You're on the path to achieving success. But don't make the mistake of thinking that setting SMART goals is enough to make them happen by themselves. If you leave them alone, they won't grow a beanstalk that magically takes you to your destination. If you sit around waiting for life to get better, it won't. If you think someone else will make your dreams happen, you're fooling yourself. Remember, only you control what happens in your life.

Change, goals, improvement—it all happens through purposeful, directed action—and that means action by **you**. Remember what we said about mental toughness being about consistent action every day? So, from now on, **every day** you need to take consistent action towards your goals.

You might have the best idea in the world, but until you make it happen, nothing will change—you won't earn any more money, get any healthier, improve your relationships, get a new job, or become an entrepreneur. Your idea will simply remain an idea. Your goal will remain just a goal. If you want to make a change, **you** have to make it happen.

Now you've discovered your path, don't let the path you've mapped out get overgrown and eventually disappear. Because that's what will happen if you don't start making actions towards your goals. And don't start walking back down the path you came from! There might be many directions we're going in, but none of them are backwards. Every day, you need to take a step forward down that path to reach your goals.

To do this, use the following steps:

1. Once you have written some big goals, choose one of those specific goals.
2. Break that goal down into smaller, more manageable steps that you can do every day.
3. Do a little of each goal every day, instead of trying to do a lot once a week.
4. Keep a track of your progress in your diary.
5. Reflect on your small wins at the end of the day.
6. Celebrate your progress each day, even if it's just a small win.
7. Be kind to yourself and stop aiming for perfection—aim for daily action.

Getting from A to Z

To get from A to Z, there's a few things you need to:

Always see your target - C

Now let me tell you one critical thing: write this down on the wall, piece of paper, set it up as a home screen on your phone, etc. It doesn't matter what you feel, or what's going on around you, you always have to **see your target**! Remember that if you can see it, you can create it; if you can feel it, you can perform it; if you can imagine it, you can achieve it.

Know your why - Y

When you know your destination, you must also know *why* you want to achieve the goals you've set, why you're doing it all. Knowing why helps you make the changes required and actually make them happen. It makes you emotionally invested in your goal. For example, if you want to earn a million dollars so you can help develop a cure for a life-threatening disease. Always keep in mind the reason for setting your goals and you won't stray from your path onto paths that jeopardise your goal.

Focus on your goal - F

If you want to be able to focus on your goal, try this exercise from a book that I personally found useful when coaching a basketball team (Karagorghis & Terry, 2010). It will help you focus on your goal and ignore distractions. Visualise that you have been asked to walk the length of a wooden plank that is 5 inches wide (12.7 cm) and 20 feet long (6m). The plank is positioned just 10 inches (25cm) off the ground. You could probably do this quite comfortably again and again without falling off—even with your hands tied behind your back! Try this in your mind's eye.

Now imagine completing the same task hands-free but with the plank raised 50 feet (15m) off the ground and positioned as a bridge between two buildings. There is no wind. It may well paralyse you with fear, but the task is the same as before. There is absolutely no difference in the physical skill required, but the additional psychological ability required is considerable.

To negotiate the 50-foot-high plank, you would need to block out thoughts of the height involved and the risk of falling, while controlling your emotions and focusing exclusively on the task at hand. In sport, the risks involved are usually far less severe than a 50-foot drop; however, your psychological reaction to even the most minor threat can be quite inhibiting. By focusing on mastering the task, you can overcome such inhibitions and perform with flair.

Moving forward with your goals

As you progress down your path, you might find that the reality is different to what you expected. Don't be alarmed. The purpose of setting goals isn't to map out the rest of your life second by second.

It's to get you moving every day in a positive direction, with purpose. Goal setting helps you build positive daily habits that move you towards long-term success.

It also helps you weed out things that aren't helping towards your goals. Setting clear goals helps you make smaller decisions, as you can quickly see whether they're in line with your long-term goals or not. For example, an athlete might think taking steroids will improve their performance. In the short-term, it might, but in the long-term, it may destroy their career and cause other health problems.

Along the way, you might find that your goals are a little different to what you thought. You'll develop knowledge that shines a light on your goals. You'll develop new methods that mean your vision changes slightly. The important thing is that you're on the path— you're going somewhere—you can just alter your course slightly. Remember, it doesn't matter if you make mistakes on your journey—if you fail from time to time. This is part of life. Maintain your mental toughness, accept your mistake, dust yourself off, and keep going.

Keep in mind this quote: "Who knows the purpose, can decide, whoever makes the decision will find peace, Who will find peace, will feel safe, Who feels safe, may think, Who thinks, can improve."

Pareto 80/20

In the business world, there is a really helpful principle called the Pareto 80/20 rule that helps in all areas of achieving your goals. You might have heard of it already. The idea is that 80% of the results or effects come from just 20% of the causes, efforts, or input. This rule works in business and in all areas of life. It particularly helps you get from A to Z, where you are now and where you want to be.

For example, 80% of your sales come from the top 20% of your customers. Your best 20% of staff create 80% of your business success. When aiming for your goals, 20% of your effort creates 80% of your progress. And so on. This means you need to identify the 20% and put your focus and efforts there, where it will create the biggest impact. These tips will help:

- Do what you do best and what you enjoy
- Implement shortcuts to save time and effort
- Delegate permission or outsource tasks you don't need to do personally
- Be selective in where you put your efforts
- Aim to be a master of a few areas instead of an average jack of all trades

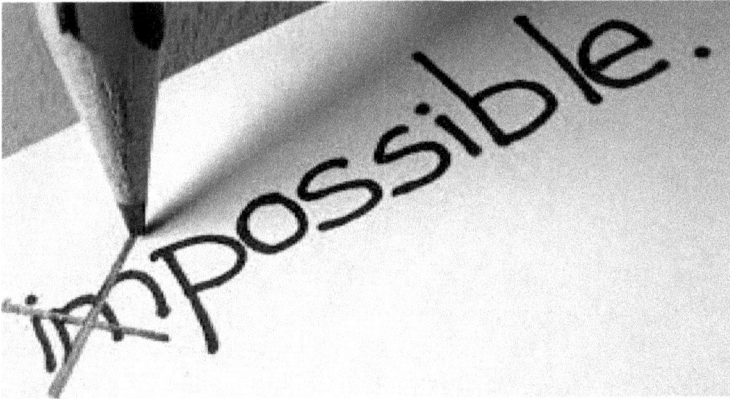

Reminder

To be successful in life, on the field, at school, or at work, you need to have a clear vision of where would you like to be—your goals. These steps will help you:

- Set up SMART goals
- Focus on your goals
- Don't be afraid of failure, success, or ridicule

- Turn big goals into small daily actions
- Use the 80/20 rule to see where to put in your effort

CHAPTER 3

Navigate Negative Feelings

"If you think you can do a thing or believe that you can't do a thing, you're right." – Henry Ford

In the last chapter, you set goals and found out how to start yourself on the right path for you in life. But inevitably, when we're pursuing our goals, negative thinking can creep in. Negative thinking is often what stops us from pursuing our dreams.

Navigating your way through negative thinking is important in developing mental toughness. This is because negative thinking stops you maintaining an attitude of being committed to positive daily action. Negative thinking affects your brain, which in turn affects your actions and behaviour. If you think negatively about yourself, you will not achieve your goals in life or improve yourself.

So, in this chapter, we'll look at how to navigate our way through negative thinking.

The effect of negativity on ourselves

You might think that negative thinking isn't anything to be concerned about. But when you're angry, upset, or thinking negatively, you're a step closer to the thing you're worrying about, or angry about, or upset about. When you think "I can't do this!", you're a step closer to *not* doing it than doing it. When you think

"I'm a terrible partner", you're a step closer to being a terrible partner. But when we turn that around, when we think positively, we're a step closer to being in a good situation. When we say, "I can do it!", we're on the way to doing it.

This is because our thinking affects our actions. Our body is heavily influenced by our mind, and so if we think negatively—if we think we can't do something—then we can't do it. By thinking negatively, we stop ourselves from achieving because we don't think we can achieve. This in turn affects our self-confidence, as we'll see in more depth in the next chapter.

On a large scale, negative thinking can lead us to feel permanently helpless. One bad situation can cause us to doubt our entire lives. One argument to doubt our whole relationship. One mistake at work to thinking we're incompetent. If we listen to all of our negative thoughts, we may even become depressed. We certainly won't have a good self-image.

What's more, when we view a situation negatively, we become nervous about it. We don't want to be in that situation, and we might avoid it and then miss out on an opportunity. But when we view it positively, we become excited, we want to be in that situation. We start to see it as an opportunity, a challenge. So, when you're starting something new, don't be nervous—be excited.

When you think positively, you embrace new situations as a challenge to overcome and learn from. You'll feel happier, and you'll get more done. You'll see the good in other things and other people, and yourself. You'll be grateful for what you have, instead of focusing on what you don't have. And you'll make the most of every opportunity that's offered to you.

The effects of negativity on others

It's not just the effect on ourselves—but our negative thinking can have an effect on other people too. Firstly, our negative thinking can actually *cause* negative situations. For example, you think you're a terrible partner, and you start to worry that your wife will leave you. Your negative thinking might cause your actions to be cold and unloving towards her. Your relationship suffers, and your negative thinking has made the situation worse. If you think positively, you can address the issues before they have a negative effect.

Negative thinking can affect your relationships. If you think negatively, the likelihood is that what you say reflects this. And if you're always talking negatively to your friends and family, you start to become a drain on other people, because they constantly have to reassure you, or try to talk you out of the negativity. The harsh reality is that negative people are no fun to be around for any length of time, so you'll notice over time that you lose friends, people don't want to spend time with you, and your loved ones lose their patience with you.

What's more, it can even affect those who don't know you. Imagine you've got a job interview and it's been you and another person. You go into the interview thinking negatively— "Why would they choose me? I'm sure the other person is better. They won't choose me. I never get chosen for anything."

Whether you know it or not, your internal negative thoughts are on display through your body language, your tone of voice, your facial expressions. In job interviews, 55% of the interviewer's decision is subconsciously based on your body language, and 38% on your tone. Without realising it, you give off negative vibes. So even if you're perfect for the job, the interviewers pick up on the negativity and they consciously or subconsciously don't choose you.

On the other hand, your competing candidate has a positive attitude and went in to the interview with positive thoughts like "I can get this job! I'm qualified for it and I'd be great for them. I know I can pass this interview!" As a result, they come across as bubbly, cheerful, and smiley. Unsurprisingly, they get the job—even if they weren't as qualified as you.

This doesn't just affect you at work, but when you're trying to attract friends or a partner. When you give off negative vibes, you don't attract the right type of person. You attract people who want to put you down to make themselves feel better. Or other negative people, who want to keep you at the same level as them. Or you attract nobody at all.

On the contrary, when you have positive thoughts and a positive attitude, you give off positive vibes. You motivate and inspire the people around you. You make friends easily, and attract the right sort of people—positive, confident people. Other people want to spend time around you, and help you when you need help. You'll find that more opportunities are offered to you.

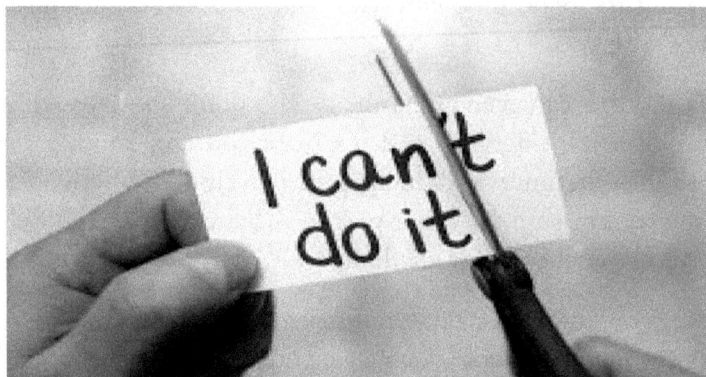

Why do we have negative thinking?

Don't berate yourself for having negative thoughts, as they are actually automatic responses from our brain. This might sound strange, but it's our mind's way of trying to protect us from a situation that might be dangerous. If our mind makes us think negatively, we might not get involved in the situation, and we'll avoid getting physically hurt, or mentally hurt. In other words, our brain is just trying to ensure our survival. Negative thoughts are a survival method. In some cases, this is actually vital, as it protects us from doing particularly reckless things that might kill us.

But that doesn't mean that all of our negative thoughts are useful or even appropriate for the circumstances. On the contrary, negative thinking becomes a fall-back habit, and before we give ourselves the chance to explore new options, our negative thinking often kicks in. The trouble is that because these thoughts come from our minds, we naturally assume that these negative thoughts are correct: *If my mind is telling me I can't do this, then I can't do it.*

In many occasions, your mind is like an overprotective parent. Of course, there is an element of risk in the situation and you may be hurt in some way, but the negative thought is nothing more than an extreme protection mechanism. There are countless dangers in the world, but it doesn't mean that we should hide indoors for our entire lives and never risk anything. So, the first thing you need to realise is that your negative thoughts are not always a realistic, appropriate assessment of the circumstances. Sometimes they are just our mind's "worst case scenario" version of events.

How to stop negative thinking

To stop negative thinking, you need to do the following:

1. Really think about the situation and try to assess the source of the thought. Is it a false alarm from your mind? Is it an over-exaggeration of the dangers? Are you trying to protect yourself from something?
2. Identify where the underlying belief comes from. For example, is it an incorrect assessment of your own abilities? Is it a negative self-belief?
3. Sometimes, talking it through with someone else will shine a light on it. Maybe writing it down will help you explore your thoughts.
4. Reframe the negative thought as a potential risk, but not a catastrophic danger that will stop you from trying to achieve your goals. Be aware of the risk and take the chance.

5. Consider how you can practically solve the problem and move on.

Don't worry if it takes a long time for you to get out of the habit of negative thinking. If you've ever tried to quit a habit, you'll know how difficult it can be. But persevere. Work your work way through the steps until you can quickly identify these unhelpful negative thoughts.

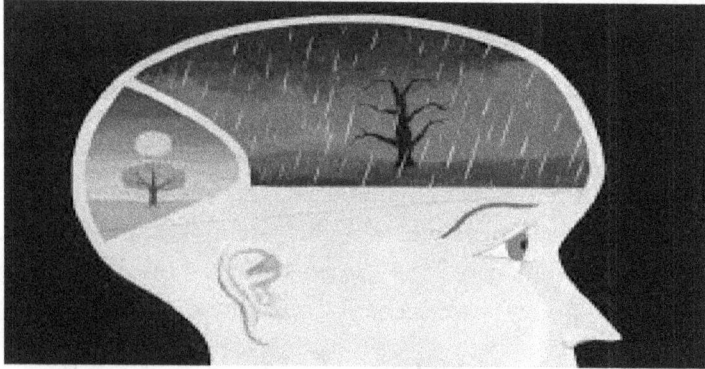

Reminder

If you think negatively, you will stop yourself from achieving your goals and dreams:

- Recognise the source of your negative thinking
- Write your thoughts down so you can understand them
- Try to swap your negative thoughts to positive thoughts
- Meditation will help you to stay positive

CHAPTER 4

Self-Confidence

"Every achiever that I have ever met says, 'My life turned around when I began to believe in me.'" - Dr Robert Schuller

In the last chapter, you learned how to deal with negative thinking. But more than that, you need to develop positive self-confidence. Unfortunately, many people misunderstand the concept of confidence. Self-confidence is a vital component in mental toughness. This is because having self-confidence gives you a better attitude.

When you're self-confident, you believe you can achieve your goals and improve yourself. As a result, self-confident people are more successful in life and enjoy life more. So in this chapter, we'll examine what confidence really is, look at the effects of having self-confidence, and discover how you can develop more of it.

Confident people

We've all met them—people who seem to snap their fingers and make good things happen in their lives, who manage to come out of every bad situation somehow better off, who always come out on top. It can be frustrating to watch, any many of us wrongly assume that these people are "lucky" or more intelligent than us, or have more money than us. Luck, intelligence, and money have nothing to do with it—it's about confidence, or more specifically, **self-confidence**. Self-confident people control their own fates. They turn challenges into opportunities. They fight through battles that knock other people down. They accept that life is difficult and they find a way through it. On the flipside, if you have no self-confidence, then minor setbacks stop you in your tracks. You're defeated by challenges. You blame your unhappy life on other people. You think life is unfair to you and you do nothing about your situation.

Take for example a footballer who experiences a nasty injury. A confident player knows they can overcome the injury and come back stronger, and they do. An unconfident player worries that the injury will end their playing career, and it takes them longer to recover. In fact, every single successful basketball player I have coached has had this vital component—self-confidence.

When it comes to achieving your goals in life, you're highly unlikely to achieve any of them if you don't have faith in yourself. A lack of self-confidence will single-handedly prevent you from achieving what you want to achieve in life, or making positive changes to your life.

What isn't self-confidence?

We often talk about needing self-confidence, but what does it really mean? First, let's talk about what self-confidence is **not**. More than any other component of mental toughness, self-confidence is the most often misunderstood. Some people mistake narcissism, superiority, ego, arrogance, and being self-centred for self-confidence. As a result, when someone is described as having "self-confidence", this is sometimes seen as a bad thing. Let's get this straight, self-confidence is not a bad thing. In fact, it's a vital thing if you want to achieve any kind of success in your life.

Self-confidence is not arrogance—it's the opposite. Self-confidence is knowing you can do something incredibly well, even the best, without having to shout it from the rooftops. Self-confident people are humble, not arrogant. It's not about assuming that everything is easily achieved, but realising the effort required and being willing to put in the hard work. On the contrary, someone who feels the need to announce their good qualities is usually lacking in confidence, rather than abundant in it.

Self-confidence is not superiority—it's the opposite. It's not thinking you're better than other people. It's knowing that you're excellent or the best at certain things and that other people are excellent and the best at other things. It's not about competing to be the best at everything, but appreciating everyone's qualities in life, including your own. People who compete to be the best in everything are not self-confident, but have a lack of confidence. Self-confident people celebrate other people's successes as well as their own.

Self-confidence is not narcissism—it's the opposite. It's not thinking you're the best at everything. It's realistically assessing and recognising your qualities and abilities and knowing that they will enable you to succeed in life. It' believing that you can improve on the things you're not so good at, with hard work and effort. It's wanting to be the best at something to improve yourself, not to show off.

Self-confidence is not self-importance or ego—it's the opposite. It's not about placing yourself above other people or only seeking your own glory. It's not about climbing the ladder to success while you trample on others. It's about wanting to be the best to improve, not in order to put other people down or succeed at the expense of others. Self-confidence is about giving your best *for* others. It's not about getting ahead in life no matter what the cost, but using your skills to make life better for everyone.

Self-confidence is not about what other people think of you—it's about what you think about yourself. As a result—**it's within your control**. If you're lacking in confidence because people have treated you badly, look inside yourself and see the real you. You've let other people's negative thoughts become your negative thoughts, your self-beliefs. Even if you've had a tough journey, and you've gone through horrible experiences, your self-confidence is up to you. Take back control of yourself, of your thoughts about yourself, of your self-beliefs.

So what is self-confidence?

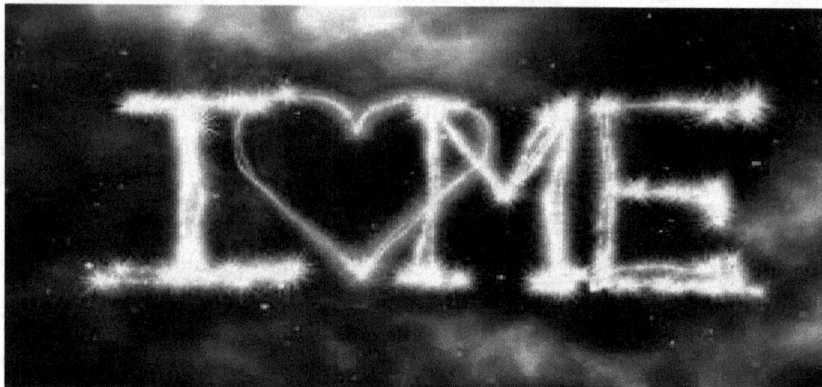

Self-confidence is believing in yourself and your abilities. It's about knowing that you as an individual have particular talents, abilities, and strengths. It is knowing what you can do, how well you can do it, and that you can improve on it. Self-confidence is:

- Recognising your own skills, qualities, and abilities, and being humble about them.
- Knowing that you have the abilities or skills to succeed in life in certain areas.
- Believing that you can improve in the areas where your skills are not as good right now.
- Understanding you have to work hard to improve, but believing that you can do it.
- Knowing that there are some things you can do better than other people and some things other people can do better than you.
- Realising that life isn't supposed to be easy, but being willing to put in the effort and hard work to succeed.

- Appreciating that other people have better skills than you in some areas and celebrating their wins too.
- Wanting to be the best at something so you can improve yourself, improve things for others, and to give others the best you have.

How do I know about self-confidence?

I know about self-confidence because I've travelled a long way from being a little boy who used to feel insecure and doubt himself most of the time, and what he thought people would think about him. I battled self-confidence issues, particularly in basketball, even though I loved it. I was confident in my studies at school, but when it came to basketball, I worried excessively and so I wasn't natural at it. I over-analysed how I played and berated myself massively when I made a mistake. When my coaches told me I had played well, I didn't believe them. I had no self-confidence in my basketball skills.

But, I listened hard to my coaches, teammates, and even famous sports stars who had succeeded. I realised I was being unfair to myself, and I more realistically assessed my abilities. I saw that I was great in some areas of playing, and not so good in others. I knew I could improve in those areas, and I worked hard to improve. I stopped letting silly mistakes get to me. I started to believe in myself—believe that I was a good player and I could succeed at basketball. In short, I developed self-confidence.

I now know that if I'm happy in my skin, that's all that matters. *I understand that I need to believe in myself before anyone else will believe in me.* Now I'm a coach, and I'll tell my players the same thing. I often tell them this famous quote from Mark Twain, "The worst loneliness is not to be comfortable with yourself." Self-confidence starts with being comfortable with yourself, in your own skin.

Why do we need confidence?

Every day, millions of people worldwide face unimaginable challenges and difficulties, but they get through them because they have self-confidence and optimism. Self-confidence leads to achievement, and enables you develop determination even when you face great difficulties. Put simply, we need confidence because we will not achieve anything in life without it.

We need confidence to face challenges and take our opportunities. If you are confident in yourself and your abilities, you have the courage to face any challenges and accept opportunities that carry a risk. You know that you have the skills, abilities, or qualities needed to succeed and achieve your goals. What's more, self-confidence means you know that if even you fail or you make a mistake, you can overcome it, learn from it, come back better, and eventually succeed. Just look at the success stories of famous people who faced and overcame extremely difficult circumstances.

We need confidence to live happily. Having self-confidence also leads us to live happier lives—not only because we achieve what we want to achieve, but because we waste less time worrying about not achieving our goals, worrying what will happen if we try to pursue them, worrying what others think about us, and worrying we will fail if we try to achieve something.

We need confidence to prepare for success. What's more, when we have confidence in our abilities, we believe we will succeed and so we plan accordingly. We know how to deal with success when it happens. On the contrary, if we don't believe we will succeed and yet we accidentally do, we didn't prepare for success and so we don't know how to deal with it and adapt accordingly. Just look at lottery winners who don't expect to win the jackpot, and when they do, they aren't prepared and often end up wasting their money and ending up back where they started. When we prepare, we feel more confident—like the opposite of a vicious circle—a happy circle, if you will.

How to build confidence – a precursor

Okay, so you see the importance of self-confidence. Before we start actually building it, you might think you're already self-confident and don't need to work on this. However, it's important to realise that most people aren't confident in every area of their life. You may be abundant in self-confidence at work, but scared to stand up to your parents. You might be confident working out at the gym, but would be terrified to speak on stage. You might be confident at home, but petrified of speaking to a stranger at a party. If we don't develop self-confidence, we miss out on opportunities in life.

You might also think you're self-confident, but perhaps you recognised some of the symptoms of "not self-confidence" mentioned earlier. Before assuming you're self-confident, check that you're not displaying arrogance, superiority, or self-importance. If you worry that you are, you need to develop true self-confidence to earn true success.

You also might think that it's not possible to develop self-confidence. It's true that some people seem naturally to be more confident than others, but like anything in life, self-confidence isn't a static limit. You **can** develop more confidence and many people have done so.

Simple steps to improve your daily self-confidence

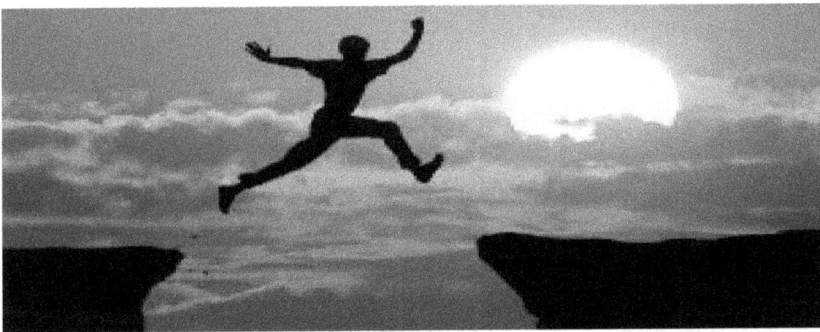

As we discussed earlier, with mental toughness, you need to make consistent daily efforts to achieve anything. And with developing self-confidence, it is no different. So, any time you encounter a situation you're worrying about or don't feel you can succeed at, follow these steps:

1. **Believe in yourself:** The most important thing in improving your self-confidence is believing in *yourself*. In any situation, you have to be kind to yourself and love yourself. Go into every situation being comfortable with yourself, in your own skin. If you treat yourself badly, judge yourself harshly, or criticise yourself in any situation, then you are depleting your self-confidence.

2. **Believe you can do it:** Think positively about the predicted outcome of the situation. People who are lack confidence expect to fail before they even start doing something, although the reality is often not as bad as the expectation. When entering any situation, believe that you can do the task at hand—that you can achieve your goals. Don't think "I can't do it" or you won't be able to do it. Instead, think "Come on, I can do this!"—pep yourself up!

3. **Counter negative thoughts:** Stop thinking negatively about the situation and worrying or doubting your abilities. When your mind presents a negative thought, counter it with a positive thought instead of giving in to the negativity. Such as countering "I can't do it" with "Oh yes I can and this is why!".

4. **Plan to succeed instead of preparing to fail:** It's tempting to go into a situation expecting to fail so you won't be disappointed when you do, saying things like "It doesn't matter if I don't pass because I know I'll fail anyway". This is a method of self-protection, but it's not a helpful one. If you go into a situation expecting to fail, you *will* fail. If you prepare to succeed, you will succeed—because you'll plan in advance to succeed.

5. **Pick yourself up when you fall down:** Inevitably, you will fail and make mistakes from time to time—it's part of life. But when you do, don't get your own back and make it

worse. To develop self-confidence, you need to be kind to yourself. Accept you made a mistake or you failed, acknowledge where you went wrong, and use it to be better next time. Get back up and keep going, instead of pushing yourself down even further.

A strategy to build self-confidence

So, you know how to build self-confidence in each individual situation, but how do you develop it over the long-term? You need a tried-and-tested strategy…

1. Fake it till you make it

This strategy is commonly known as "fake it till you make it", and was first suggested by Dale Carnegie, author of the famous book *How to Win Friends and Influence People.* He suggested that if you act the way you want to be, you will become what you want to be.

One way to develop self-confidence is in your movements. If you watch confident people, they walk straight and tall (no matter how physically tall they are), they hold their heads high, and smile or make eye contact. People who are not confident slouch, hang their heads, and don't make eye contact with others. But more than just watching them—mimic their movements. It sounds crazy, but by walking tall, you start to *feel* better.

If you don't believe me, try it for yourself. Try purposefully and actively walking both ways and see how you feel after both. I guarantee you'll feel better after walking tall. So, from now on, I want you to make yourself walk tall every day, hold yourself up straight, make eye contact and smile at people—even if you feel like you don't want to. The reaction you get might surprise you.

2. Look at your thinking

While you're faking it outwardly, you also need to look inwardly to locate the cause of your lack of self-confidence and fix the problem. Think of it this way, if your washing machine is broken, what do you do? You hire someone who knows about washing machines to take it apart and find the source of problem and you fix it. (Before you say buy a new one, you can't buy a new self!) You are the expert on yourself, so you need to look inside, figure out what's going wrong, and then work on fixing it.

An easy way to start is by taking note of what you think about on a day-to-day basis. Be honest with yourself about what you're thinking. Are you constantly thinking negative thoughts? Are you worrying all the time? Are you angry or upset a lot? If you are—is it any wonder that you're not happy in life? That you're not achieving what you want to? As Earl Nightingale once said, "Every one of us is the sum total of his own thoughts".

If you want anything to change in your life, you have to change your thinking first. Much research on self-confidence has demonstrated that *how you think* plays the most important role in success. It's not what you do—it's how you think about it. So work on purposefully and actively changing your thinking. Instead of focusing on failure, focus on success. Instead of worrying about what might go wrong, think of ways to ensure it goes right. Instead of thinking about the risks, think about what could go right. Instead of preparing yourself to fail, plan to win. Fill your mind with thoughts of what you want to achieve, and how you can achieve it.

Don't let your thoughts control you—you control them. Don't let your mind run away with you, with your dreams and goals. Take control of your thoughts and every time you have a negative thought—fight back with a positive one. Every time your mind tells you that you can't do something, tell it you can, figure out how, and make it happen.

3. Embrace lifelong learning

One major way to improve your confidence is through learning. We live in an ever-changing world, so we can't make the mistake of thinking that we can stay still. We need to keep working on and improving ourselves, practicing and developing our skills. Self-confidence is often described as being like a knife that you need to sharpen every so often to keep it cutting well. So if we want lifelong self-confidence, we need to embrace a mindset of *forever learning*.

As society around us changes rapidly, with new inventions and developments in science and technology, we need to go with the trend of change in order to adapt to our new environment. Think of it this way—as we encounter new situations or new objects, our confidence diminishes because we lack knowledge of this new thing. By learning, we gain knowledge and skills that enable us to deal with new things, and thus we maintain our confidence over time.

Learning also helps us overcome failures or losses. For instance, say you have lost the championship game. You're feeling miserable, upset, angry even—and your self-confidence is knocked. By learning, by gaining knowledge and skills, you will have more self-confidence and will perform better next time. There is a common phrase that "if a person has self-confidence, they have won half the battle."

4. Become a master at your strengths

Sometimes, your lack of self-confidence can be a result of not recognising your own skills and abilities. It's important that you have a realistic view of yourself in order to develop self-confidence. So, get a notepad and write down everything good about you—your skills, qualities, and abilities, anything you're good at.

An easy way to do this is think about what people have complimented you on or thanked you for in the past. Then, become a master of your strengths by picking a few of these good points to improve on. When you see that you can improve on the things you're already good at, it'll be easier to improve in the areas you're not currently as good at.

5. Model confidence in others

When you're trying to develop self-confidence, you need to model the actions and thoughts of positive, confident people. If you surround yourself with other negative people, they will only bring you down further. It can help to talk to confident, positive people, as can often shine a light on you being unnecessarily harsh to yourself, or misjudging your abilities. They can help put things into perspective for you, and make you realise you've been putting yourself down. Watch confident people in action and in videos. Read books by successful, confident people. Be inspired by those who are confident and model yourself on them. To clarify, this doesn't mean seeking self-validation from others, as self-confidence doesn't come from others, but getting a realistic view of yourself.

6. Establish realistic objectives

Often, our self-confidence is affected because we have unrealistic objectives in life. You need to understand your abilities and build realistic goals around them. This means setting goals that are achievable—not too high nor low. If you have extremely high standards or expectations for yourself, you will be disappointed. If your goals are unrealistically high, you don't reach them, and it will knock your self-confidence. Realise that nobody is perfect, and you can't be good at everything.

In contrast, setting your standards too low may cause over-confidence, as you will be so comfortable achieving your goals that you may become arrogant or mistakenly judge your own abilities. Your goals should be challenging, but not impossible.

7. Never give up.

Often, we have low self-confidence because we've given up too quickly. We have a go at something, we can't do it the first or second time, so we assume we're doomed to never do that thing. This is known as a defeatist attitude. We stop trying, we give up, we say "It's too hard" or "I tried and I can't do it!". First, realise that life is a long game, and it might take years to win. Success takes time and effort. So when you don't get it right first time, learn from your mistakes and keep going until you do succeed. Keep learning, improving, developing until you do succeed.

Never give up on your goals. Never throw in the towel.

Self-confidence in sports

If you play a sport, you're often likely to come across situations where self-confidence is a vital factor in your success, particularly in elite sports, where you regularly face intense competition. I've seen this first-hand many times as a basketball coach. It's known as "performance anxiety", and almost all athletes experience it from time to time.

You start to think negatively and think that you'll lose. You start to worry what might happen if you don't win, and put yourself under pressure. You worry about the effect of the outcome on your career, or your family, or your income. The trouble with performance anxiety is that your body reacts physically to this, and you start to suffer performance loss as a result.

So when you start to think like that, how do you quell the fear of these pressure thoughts? Firstly, you need to put the situation into perspective. Ask yourself questions like:

- If I don't win this game, will I lose my family, friends, or my home?
- Will I end up begging on the street?

This will take the importance off the upcoming match or event. Pressure thoughts are not reality—one loss is not the end of your career, and it certainly won't result in you losing your friends and family.

As a coach, I help athletes get over performance anxiety by encouraging them to embrace their painful emotions. They need to understand that all emotions are trying to tell them something— they are a signal to get us to act on something that it is important to us.

For example, one of my best basketball players suddenly started to make silly mistakes and get anxious during a game. He normally averaged at least 15 points a game, but in this game, he didn't score any. I realised that when the game started, his ex-girlfriend appeared with her new boyfriend and this distracted him so much that he couldn't stay calm and focused. When he realised this, he dealt with the emotions and managed to control them. During the next game, he played well again as he focused only on the court and the next play.

In sport, as well as each player being confident in their own abilities, they must also be confident in their teammates, and they must work together to ensure success. It's the same in an office or any workplace. This means they need to communicate, help each other overcome difficult times, and work together. It's not a competition. Mental toughness displayed as self-confidence isn't just about helping yourself but helping others. Being tough isn't about pushing people down but helping them back up.

Reminder

A self-confident person:

- Is comfortable in their own skin and believes in themselves and their abilities, skills, and qualities.
- Has a realistic view of themselves, sets realistic objectives, and strives to improve in areas they are not so good at.
- Accepts their mistakes, learns from errors and failures, and never gives up.
- Faces challenges, takes opportunities, and knows they can overcome difficulties.
- Doesn't worry about what might happen and instead plans for success.
- Is humble, wants to see others succeed, and recognises the skills and qualities of others.
- Embraces lifelong learning, moves with the times, and keeps developing.
- Surrounds themselves with other confident people and models successful people.
- Wants to improve themselves to give their best for others.

CHAPTER 5

Concentration

"If you can keep playing tennis when somebody is shooting a gun down the street, that's concentration." – Serena Williams

To develop mental toughness, you need the right skills and abilities, and one of those is the ability to concentrate on one thing. Concentration is vital to mental toughness. This is because mental toughness is being committed to consistent daily action. To do, you need the ability to focus your attention on a single thought or subject and not get distracted from your goals. Developing this skill is useful in many parts of your life, enabling you to focus on the task at hand, either at work, on the field, or at home.

So, in this chapter, we'll look at the importance of concentration in developing mental toughness. I'll also show you some techniques to help you improve your concentration so you can become mentally tougher.

The importance of concentration

We might think we know what concentration is, but let's agree on a definition before we go any further. Concentration is our capacity or ability to focus on just one subject, object, or thought at one time, and to reject any other disconnected thoughts, emotions, or sensations from our mind. It means taking your mind off numerous things and putting all of your attention on one given thing. In other words, you are focusing on just **one thing.** More than that, it is about being in the present moment, in the here and now.

Concentration is vital for mentally tough people as it enables them to focus on the most important things, and ignore the distractions or other stimuli. Consider a sprinter about to start a 100-meter gold medal race. If they don't have effective concentration skills, they'll get distracted by the noise of the crowd, the other athletes preparing, or the heat of the day—rather than focusing on the race.

It's easy to see how concentration is vital for performance in sports, but it's also vital in other high-pressure situations. Imagine presenting at a conference in front of hundreds of people, and instead of concentrating on your presentation, you're focused on someone loudly eating crisps on the front row, or someone coughing at the back of the room.

You see, when you break your concentration for a moment, it opens the door to negative thoughts. Fear and doubt sneak in, and then you struggle to regain your focus, your concentration slips, and then you start to get annoyed with yourself and react emotionally. You lose the race, or you lose your audience.

But it's not just in these high-pressure situations that concentration is important. Think about when you were setting your goals. You can't set goals if you can't focus on what you want. In fact, what often stops people from setting clear goals is that they struggle to focus on what they actually want, and instead they get distracted. Sometimes, the only difference between someone who achieves something and someone who doesn't is the former's ability to concentrate on their given task.

Some of the most influential people of our times, such as Bill Gates and Steve Jobs, the inventors of Microsoft and Apple, were renowned for possessing incredible skills in concentration. Though ironically, their inventions mean it's particularly easy for us to get distracted these days! In our modern age of smartphones, we're often trying to focus on a task, but we keep getting emails or

Facebook notifications pop up. So being able to concentrate is an essential ability if you want to survive the demands of the modern age.

Train your brain to concentrate

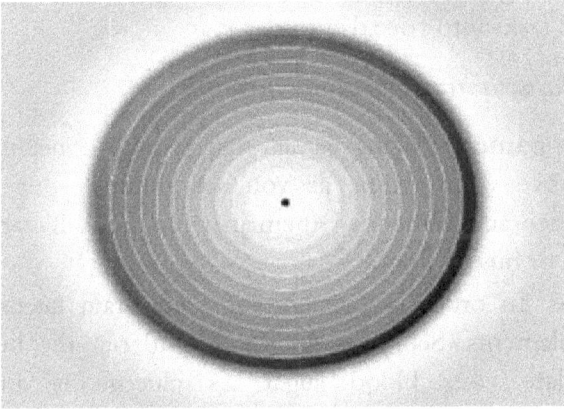

The great news is you can train yourself to refocus your attention when it slips. The easiest way to train yourself in concentration is practising meditation. This can be as simple as lying down away from distractions, shutting your eyes for 10 minutes, and focusing on just one thing whilst trying to shut out your other thoughts. An easy one to start with is focusing on your breathing—the movement of your chest going up and down. Not only will this help you train your mind to focus on one thing, but practicing your breathing also helps you reduce your anxiety in stressful, high-pressure situations.

This might sound time-consuming, and it certainly won't happen overnight, but it's absolutely worth doing, and in the long term, it will improve your concentration skills. You might even notice an improved ability to concentrate in just a short space of time.

Current research shows that we can improve our brain's ability to perform functions such as concentration. When we gain knowledge, our mind's associations and neurones are subject to change and improvement. Our minds are not static things stuck at a certain skill level and unable to improve. We can always improve, but to do so, we need to turn our knowledge into practical action and keep using our new skills.

You guessed it—we need to make consistent, practical actions every day to develop concentration, just like with mental toughness. So, to start improving your concentration, you can have a go at fitting these small tasks into your day-to-day plan.

Daily actions to improve concentration

- **Play games**: Playing games that require concentration can improve your ability, as you are putting your skills into practice and cementing them in your brain. Try this on the train or bus to work.
- **Food**: In order to concentrate, your brain needs the right supplements. See your doctor to find out the best way to regulate your blood sugar, as glucose is an essential supplement for your mind.
- **Contemplate**: Try to ponder twice every day, around 5 minutes in the morning and 5 minutes at night.
- **Sleep and rest**: It's crucial to get a sufficient sleep and relaxation time, because you'll struggle to concentrate otherwise.
- **Reward yourself**: If your task at hand isn't fun but needs to be done, then reward yourself when you've done it as this will improve your motivation. Try not to make the reward unhealthy though.
- **Avoid distractions**: Turn off loud, distracting noises. If you're working somewhere noisy, try to move somewhere quiet. If you can't move elsewhere, try listening to soft, instrumental music with headphones.
- **Set a schedule:** The human brain likes order, so set a daily schedule and do the same tasks at the same time every day.
- **Keep it separate:** Keep your work and home life separate, so don't practice your hobbies in your relaxation room, or try to relax where you work.

- **Set the mood:** This may sound odd, but colours affect the human mind in different ways! According to a recent study, green light improves concentration. So try buying some green bulbs.
- **Take breaks:** Take regular short breaks during the day, so you can concentrate when you need to.

Strategies to learn and maintain concentration

As well as these daily habits to improve concentration, you can also implement these wider strategies:

1. **Visualisation:** This means vividly imagining where you want to be, what you want to do, and so on—*before* the situation happens. It might be playing out a presentation you have at work tomorrow, or an exam you have to take. The important thing is visualising the whole situation exactly as you want it to play out. Visualise your success. Imagine yourself winning. Doing this will also improve your self-confidence.

2. **Get present:** Focus on the present moment and centre your attention on what your senses are experiencing right now. Fear doesn't exist in the present moment.

3. **Use mantras:** Find a mantra or phrase that becomes a trigger for you. These words will help you to stay focused, such as "I can do this", "This is my time", or "I never give up".

4. **Let it go:** To concentrate, you need to forget the mistake you just made, or made in the past. Make a habit of forgiving yourself out loud when you make a mistake. Mistakes and failures are part of life, so quickly forgive yourself and move on.

5. **Practice focusing:** Practise your ability to focus a few times a day by picking up an item and timing how long you can concentrate on it without other thoughts creeping in. Your concentration is like a muscle that gets stronger as you train.

You get better and better by working on it, and then it becomes a habit.

Learning to concentrate through meditation

One great way to learn to concentrate is through meditation. There's a lot of misconceptions about meditation, and it certain won't magically take away all the bad bits of your character or your life. It won't turn you into a pleasant or calm person overnight, or even forever. But it will help you on your journey. For me, it helps me feel okay with the imperfect and unsatisfactory truth of being a human.

Meditation and mindfulness teach us to remain present in awkward moments, without needing to change them. Being able to sit still when you're experiencing pain or discomfort is incredibly liberating when you realise that it won't kill you. The stillness of meditation creates distance between you and your thoughts, diminishing their power over you. It will also help you overcome negative thoughts in the long run, so why not try it?

If you don't know how to start, try focusing on a single object, such as a candle flame, an affirmation, or your breathing. It will be difficult at first and you will get distracted, but try to stay in the moment and just focus on that one thing. Over time, it will get easier to focus.

Concentration for sportspeople

Concentration is particularly vital if you're an athlete, as you'll often find yourself in high-pressure situations where you need to focus. Follow the example of your sporting heroes to improve your concentration. If you watch the best sports stars, they focus on the important things and maintain this focus over a sustained period of time. Despite this narrow focus, they are still aware of the situation, and they can shift their focus when they need to in order to perform at their best.

Cricketer Garfield Sobers, the great West Indies bowler, famously described concentration as "a shower—you don't turn the tap on until you want to take a shower. You don't walk out of the shower and leave it running. You turn it off and turn on when has to be fresh and ready when you need it." In other words, successful athletes learn techniques to concentrate their minds and have task-oriented focus in close, competitive situations.

The importance of concentration in sport cannot be understated. It can be the difference between winning and losing, crossing the line first or 0.3 seconds later. There are many successful athletes out there, and even amateurs, whose physical ability is very similar to the best players in the world, yet they don't reach the same level of success. The difference is their ability to concentrate and control their attention. Those highly successful players are the ones who can shut out distractions.

Tips to effectively concentrate in sports

- Put in deliberate, mental discipline and intentional effort.
- Prepare to concentrate, rather than standing around and waiting for it to occur.
- Adopt a "just do it" mindset.
- Discuss, think through, and rehearse strategies beforehand.
- Focus on only one thought at a time.
- Concentrate on actions that are accurate, relevant, and under your control.
- Stay in the moment—don't think about how your favourite NBA team is doing.
- Be ready to re-focus as focus can be broken at any time.
- Be prepared for auditory distractions such as crowd noise, aeroplanes flying overhead, or public announcement systems.
- Be prepared for visual distractions such as flags waving or flashes from cameras.

- Focus on the process, such as technique and proficiency, rather than the outcome.

Reminder

To help you improve your concentration and increase your focus, you need to:

- Forget mistakes you've just made and instead focus on the present.
- Look after your health—get sufficient rest and relaxation, and eat healthily.
- Try meditation to improve your focus.
- Remove noise or distractions, and listen to relaxing music.
- Focus on one thought at a time—don't try to multitask.

CHAPTER 6

Discipline

"I hated every minute of training, but I said, 'Don't quit. Suffer now and live the rest of your life as a champion.'" - Muhammad Ali

When we hear the word "discipline", we often think it's a bad thing, and we react negatively. But actually, discipline is vital in developing mental toughness. The ability to be disciplined will help you solve life's problems. It's also something that many of us lack.

Discipline is a vital component in developing mental toughness. This is because mental toughness is being committed to consistent daily action, and this requires a huge amount of discipline as some days you just won't feel like doing it. On those days, you need the ability to be disciplined so you can stay on track, make yourself work towards your goals when you feel demotivated, and fight against your emotions when they are distracting you.

So, in this chapter, we'll look at the importance of discipline and how to become more self-disciplined to achieve our goals.

How do I become more disciplined?

There are no shortcuts in life to achieve your goals. If you don't want to repeat the same cycle over and over again, like a washing machine, then you must apply self-discipline. With self-discipline, you can begin to reverse the effects of your negative thoughts and slowly become the captain of your own life.

Discipline is one of the main foundations of success. Any famous person who has succeeded in life probably had a problem with discipline at the start. But they developed discipline, and they succeeded. We also have the ability to learn discipline. Just don't expect that you'll have a natural talent for it at the start.

At some point, you've probably experienced a lack of discipline. For example, maybe you had to write a budget plan at work. For the first few days, you probably didn't have the motivation to do anything with it. Then you started doing it at the last minute. With discipline, you'll start it straight away. If you had more discipline in aiming for your goals, you would be closer to achieving them right now. So, as you can see, discipline is one of the essential tools in succeeding at anything in life.

To start developing discipline, pick a goal that you want to be more disciplined in. For example, better nutrition, better results at school, a better position at work, or on your sports team. Here are four ways you can become more disciplined:

1. Be more emotionally engaged in your dream.

Sometimes it's hard to stay invested in our goal and be disciplined when we're tempted to do other things. Why work on our dreams when we could watch TV or lie on the sofa or surf the internet right? There will be time for our goals later, right? But when you're emotionally engaged in your dream, you know the reason you're doing it and this reason is a strong motivating factor in being disciplined.

For example, when I was learning English in Scotland, it was tempting to spend my days off just lying in bed and relaxing. But I knew that I really wanted to learn English because I wanted to improve myself and open a world of opportunities available to English speakers. So, I made myself study every day.

So, when you're feeling lazy or demotivated, you can force yourself back to being disciplined by reminding yourself of the motivating factor behind your goals. After all, it's easier to get off the sofa and make yourself do something if you have a great reason pushing you forward.

2. Control your chaotic life.

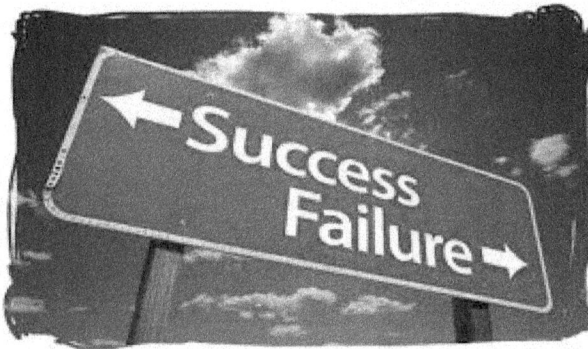

You need to be prepared for the challenges of your daily life, so you can keep sight of your aims. Start a daily routine every morning, which over time will become a habit. When you have a routine, it brings order to the chaos. This will help you ensure you have time to work on your goals rather than always playing catch up with them.

When planning your daily routine, consider how you can be more efficient and put yourself and your priorities in first place. Write down in your notebook what you need to achieve to be satisfied with your day. When you get up, don't waste time checking social media. First, do the things that are most important to you, and don't waste time on things that are not relevant. Don't let useless things waste your time every day. Then make sure you do your daily tasks.

When you postpone them, often you'll never finish them thoroughly. Do not give yourself a reason for excuses.

3. Book time for the most important things.

Reserve blocks of time during the day when you only work with full concentration on a given task. Let's say I spend 20 minutes before breakfast, 20 minutes during the day, and 20 minutes before dinner on these tasks. For those 20 minutes, I concentrate fully. After a few days of systematic work 20 minutes, three times a day, discipline will be in my blood. Write a reminder in your notebook or phone when you will spend these three 20 minutes every day on your daily tasks.

4. Reward yourself.

Celebrate small successes. This is crucial. Why is it crucial? If we do something regularly every day and we get no positive reaction, then our brain will pull us away from it. Our brain likes pleasure—that's why it's so hard to get up in the morning. Give yourself a reward. For instance, when I wrote a chapter of this book, I went for a dinner to a new restaurant or bought a small gift for myself. Rewards help you feel more satisfied and proud of what you did, and this helps to build discipline.

Discipline and pleasure must be connected in your mind, as then discipline becomes pleasant to you. When you're disciplined, you get nearer to your goal, and you understand the purpose of what you're doing every day. If you keep practising these four points, you'll quickly see how discipline change you for the better. Eventually, it will come naturally, rather than feeling like a chore, and you'll start to see the results of your efforts in moving closer your goals.

Reminder

Self-discipline is one of the important ingredients of success. It expresses itself in a variety of ways:

- Perseverance and self-control.
- The ability not to give up, despite failure and setbacks.
- The ability to resist distractions or temptations.
- Trying over and again, until you accomplish what you set out to do.

CHAPTER 7

The Ability To Say "NO"

"The difference between successful people and really successful people is that really successful people say no to almost everything." Warren Buffet

In the last chapter, you saw the importance of discipline in order to develop mental toughness. This involves the ability to say "no" when necessary. I know it can be very difficult to say "no", especially to friends and family.

The ability to say "no" is important in mental toughness. This is because mental toughness means being committed to consistent daily action. If you have no time for your goals, how can you be committed to working on them every day? If you're constantly busy and tired, you won't be productive or have time for your goals or yourself. To have time for your goals and the energy to work on them, you need to be able to say "no" to some things.

So, in this chapter, we'll look at when you need to say "no" and *how* to say it.

The effect of people pleasing

In life, many of us are "people pleasers" and by that I mean we struggle to say "no". Whether it's saying "no" to offering someone help when we're overworked already, saying "no" to an event we don't really want to go to, saying "no" to a pushy salesperson offering us something we don't need, or saying to the waiter "no, everything is not okay with my meal. It's undercooked." We've probably all been there, where we've said yes just to please people when inside we're shouting NOOOOOOOOOOOOO!

I'll admit, I used to be terrible at saying "no" to people. I didn't want to upset anyone, and I liked seeing the happy look on someone's face when I said "yes". I didn't want to seem rude, unkind, or unhelpful. I didn't want to let people down, disappoint them, or upset them. And I was convinced this would happen if I said "no". Most of the time, when we don't want to say "no" to people, it's because we're worried what they'll think about us.

Saying "yes" to everything was fine to an extent, as long as I could shift some priorities to help out, miss a workout to go to the event, afford to buy the item, or not eat the bad food. But as I got older, and my priorities grew and grew, I realised that saying "yes" all the time wasn't feasible. Suddenly, I had a wife to put first, a basketball team to coach, and a new job in management to work hard at. I didn't have time or money to waste on saying "yes" to everything.

By saying yes to extra work, I was sprinting from the office to basketball coaching. By agreeing to drink with a friend who was lonely, I was staying up late to squeeze in time with my wife, then waking up tired for work. By agreeing to walk a friend's dog, I was missing a morning gym session. I was exhausted and overstretched. You get the picture. The trouble is, we get asked to do more things all the time, but our schedule often doesn't allow it all.

One of the first things to go is our self-care. We sacrifice the gym for something extra, grab unhealthy food because we're running late from trying to fit everything in, and we make no time for relaxation before bed. We end up tired, ineffective, and stretched too thin. We don't offer the best of ourselves to anyone, including ourselves. So, what started out as us not wanting to let anyone down inevitably ends up with us getting ill and being unable to help anyone. We get miserable and grouchy.

What's more, we don't have time to work on our dreams and goals. We lose our consistent daily actions. We forget to improve ourselves. We don't strive for anything more because we don't have time. We don't even have time to consider where we're going wrong. If you recognise any of this, STOP RIGHT NOW. Start saying "no" and getting your time back so you can work on yourself, develop mental toughness, and achieve your goals.

Why do we say "yes"?

So why do we often feel that we have to say "yes"? Firstly, we're taught as children that it's polite to say "yes". "Did you like your dinner?" Yes. "Do you like your present?" Yes.

Then, when we get friends, we say "yes" because it makes us popular. Like saying "yes" to hanging out with our friends every night or going to every party instead of doing our homework.

When we start work, we say "yes" so our manager will like us, so our colleagues will like us. "Do you want to do overtime?" Yes. "Would anyone like extra responsibilities?" Yes.

We don't want to be rude, unpopular, or disliked. So, we get into the habit of saying "yes" when we want to say "no". As humans, we naturally don't want to be rejected by other people, so we avoid this rejection by always saying "yes".

But ultimately, life isn't about doing things we don't want to do in order to be liked by other people. When you say "no" to please others, you choose them over yourself—you diminish your self-worth. Your self-worth depends on you, not on how much you do to please others. There comes a time when you have to stop doing things to please others, and do what's right for you.

Top 10 tips to start saying "no"

1. **Start with "maybe".** If we start with something small, like saying "maybe", then we get into the habit of not saying "yes" to everything. But don't say "maybe" if you really mean "no" as it will just cause more stress in the meantime. So...

2. **Get it over with quickly.** Sometimes, we build up saying "no" in our heads until we've avoided it so long that it becomes too late and we end up doing it anyway. Get it over with as soon as the request comes in—this means less time worrying about saying it later or resenting the person for something you didn't want to do.

3. **Practise saying "no".** Imagine being asked to do something and rehearsing how you will say "no". The more you say it, the easier it gets over time.

4. **Start small.** Start saying "no" to smaller requests before trying to say "no" to the big ones.

5. **Practice saying "no" to strangers.** Before saying "no" to loved ones, practise saying "no" to strangers, such as a salesman trying to sell you something you don't need.

6. **Have a reason for saying "no".** It's hard to say "no" without a reason, so try saying "no, I can't this time as I have to do x instead."

7. **Don't lie about the reason.** If you lie about your reason for saying "no", you'll only end up feeling guilty. Be honest if you give a reason and your friends will understand this better.

8. **Focus on the benefits of saying "no".** Instead of focusing on the negative, such as upsetting someone, focus on the benefit of taking care of yourself so you're more effective.

9. **Don't be sorry, be polite.** Say "thanks for the offer but..." rather than "I'm so sorry, I can't...". Don't feel you need to apologise for not having time to do something.

10. **Think about your answer.** If you answer too quickly, it can sound like you're rejecting the person. Check your calendar and give a measured answer.

Develop time management rules

Saying "no" is easier when you have rules to check the request against. That way, your response isn't an emotional response, but a structured one. It's "my schedule doesn't allow it" rather than "I personally don't want to".

To do this, plan out your week in advance allowing for work, the gym, relaxation, sleep, family time, and working on your goals— basically, anything in your consistent daily actions plan that you developed earlier. When you've done this, there should be gaps in your calendar. If there are no gaps, you need to go back and start phasing out somethings you've already agreed to!

Then, based on your available time, set some rules. For example:

- I have three free nights a week, so I can only plan something on one of them. One is for my wife. One is for my self-development.
- I am committed to being healthier, so I won't go out for food or drinks this month.
- I have two free mornings before work, so I can go out for coffee with a friend one morning.

This way, when someone asks you to do something, you can look at your calendar and instantly see whether you're free. If you are free, you can check whether your rules allow it.

Saying "no" to a friend or loved one

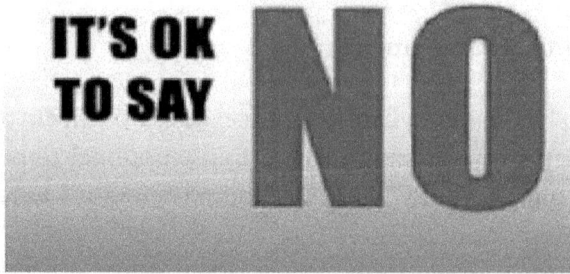

Sometimes, we're okay saying "no" to strangers, but we always give into friends or family because we're scared of upsetting them and ruining the friendship or relationship. The trouble with doing this is that if we always say "yes", they come to expect it, and suddenly we have no free time at all. We have to learn to say "no" to friends and family, otherwise when they really need us, we'll be too exhausted to help them.

There are two ways to approach this. If they're a close friend or family member, explain your situation to them. Tell them how overstretched you are. Friends and loved ones will understand when you're stretched too thin or you're committed to something else. If they're upset by your refusal after you've explained the circumstances, then they're not being a good friend.

The other approach is to not explain the situation in detail and simply say "I have other plans" or "I can't right now". This approach is often best for distant friends or your wider circle, as they don't need to know your particular situation right now. Don't feel obliged to give everyone the details of your life.

To do this, you need to realise there is nothing wrong with saying "no". There is nothing bad about saying "no" to ensure your own wellbeing and happiness. After all, you can't help anyone else if you don't help yourself first. Think of this way—when you're on a plane, the safety instructions are always to fit your own oxygen mask first in an emergency before helping anyone else fit theirs.

People think they should fit their child's mask first, but if they don't fit their own mask first, they won't be able to help their child and both will suffer.

If you want to succeed at your goals, achieve your dreams, and develop mental toughness, you have to be able to say "no". When you say "no", you are giving sufficient time to your priorities. You are staying true to yourself. You don't need to feel bad, because you are doing the right thing for you.

Reminder

There is nothing wrong with saying no:

- If you don't want to do something, or don't have time.
- If saying "yes" means you are getting burnt out or don't time to work on your goals.
- Saying "no" is not selfish. Saying "no" is not rude. Saying "no" is not wrong.
- Saying "no" to others is saying "yes" to yourself—to your health and to your goals.
- Saying "no" leads to a better life balance and a more harmonious existence.

CHAPTER 8

Openness To Change

"We can change who we are. We can improve ourselves in various ways, and we can give ourselves possibilities" - James Heckman

In the previous section, you developed the skills and abilities required for mental toughness. When you have the skills required, you need to use them to approach life in the right way. In this section, you'll see the approaches required for mental toughness.

One of these key approaches is being open to change. Openness to change is another vital part of mental toughness. This is because mental toughness is having the right attitude to self-improvement. If you're not open to change, you don't move forward in life—you just stay where you are and never improve yourself or your circumstances.

If you're open to change, you come up with new ideas, discover new experiences, and enjoy new situations, which all enables you to gain success and achieve your goals. So, in this chapter, you'll see the importance of being open to change, and you'll discover how to open yourself up.

What does it mean to be open to change?

As humans, we naturally like to think we're open to change. But in reality, when we're in a situation that requires change, we feel scared or angry. We often react badly to change, whether it's a small change like our favourite TV show being cancelled, or a big change like our company being restructured.

Firstly, being open to change doesn't mean loving every change that takes place, but understanding that change is an essential part of life, and that we need to continually adapt and grow to succeed. It's being able to take on board new information and use it to improve yourself. If you're closed to new ideas, you'll never improve or achieve your goals. You need to step outside your comfort zone.

If you look at successful people in life, they aren't afraid of change. In fact, they embrace change. They see change as an opportunity for success. They step out of their comfort zone. They learn new skills, become more flexible, and more agile, and are often more adaptable than they thought they could be. In turn, they become more confident in themselves and their ability to be successful.

Why are we not open to change?

There are many reasons we might be closed to change, but these are some of the common ones:

Ego: Often, the reason we're not open to change is because our ego tells us that we know best. Nobody else could know better than us. For example, say your goal is to open your business in five new markets that are turning a profit in the next 18 months. You open the businesses but they don't seem to be turning a profit. Someone suggests advertising in a different way to suit the culture of the new places, but you're not open to changing your advertising methods, you think you know advertising best, so you ignore the advice. You don't turn a profit and end up closing the new business and making a loss.

Living in the past: Another reason we're often closed to change is because we're living in the past, instead of the present. This means you never move forward. We think this is the way it's always been done and this is the way it should stay. But life doesn't stay till. Time is always moving on. And we need to move with it. For example, our company implements a new software system and we have to learn it. We think what was wrong with paper and pen? But the world has moved on and technology improves efficiency, freeing up time for other useful tasks. So, we need to learn the new task.

Lack of self-confidence: Another common reason is fear and lack of self-confidence. We're worried we don't have the skills or abilities to deal with the change. For example, your company is being restructured, and you're worried about losing the job you've had for years. But if you have self-confidence and positive thinking, you'll see it as an opportunity to do something new—develop new skills, try out a new role, or even make the leap to being an entrepreneur instead.

All of this can lead to depression, a mid-life crisis, lack of satisfaction with your life, and not achieving your goals. When your mind is closed, you're limiting your potential in life, because you're closed to new ideas or information.

What do I know about being open to change?

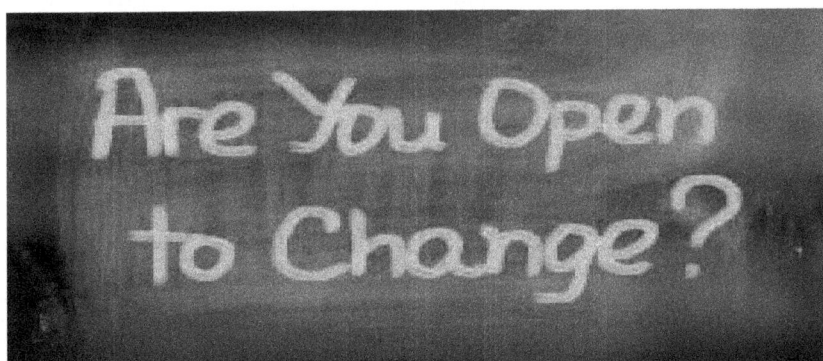

As I mentioned earlier, I grew up in Poland during difficult times. As a teenager, I thought very negatively and had self-confidence issues. I didn't like myself and I doubted my own abilities. I didn't think I'd succeed at anything in life. When people suggested new ideas to me that might have helped me, I rejected them because my mind was closed. But I wanted to learn about myself, stand on my own two feet, and open the doors to the new opportunities.

Then one day, I realised I was getting nowhere with my own ideas, and I needed to open my mind to new ideas if I wanted to improve and make changes. Suddenly, things started to improve. I listened harder and developed more new ideas. I embraced a mindset of being open to change all the time. I tried new things, and I kept trying different things until something worked.

One suggestion I listened to was going travelling. As someone with low self-confidence, and who was closed-minded, travelling wasn't something I'd considered, but it was a great idea. So, I decided to open my mind and go to Scotland and then to England. Although many people say they want to travel, many don't—and this is because travel requires you to be constantly open to change. Travel means saying goodbye to the known and experiencing a new culture, language, food, customs, and people. When people go travelling, they sometimes experience culture shock, and they feel "homesick", missing the familiar instead of embracing the change.

I learned to embrace this change, because it helped me learn more about myself, how to survive in different circumstances, and how to communicate with different people. I made great friends while travelling, and listened to their different experiences. It's an often-said cliché that travel opens your mind, but from experience, I've seen that this is true.

When I opened my mind, it ensured that I didn't let my ego limit my growth. As a result, I learned to speak English, coach basketball, pass advanced exams at the Management Academy, write a book, meet Kobe Bryant and Jimmy Connors, and help others to succeed. When your mind is open, your life will be better because you'll be open to trying new things that you haven't tried before. If your mind is closed, your life won't change.

How to open your mind

To clarify, I'm not saying you need to go travelling to open your mind. It's one way, but it's not the only way. Say you want to earn more money. If you don't believe that you can make more, then you never will because your mind is limited and closed to new ideas and projects that might make you earn more. Instead, you'll stay working in the same job, profession, or company and expect something to change by magic.

First you need to realise that you don't have all of the information and ideas that are out there, so you can always learn more about earning more. When someone presents an idea of how to earn more, listen to them and take the ideas on board. Rather than rejecting the ideas, mull them over and think whether you could make them happen. Try the suggestions and see what works for you. Embrace new money-making opportunities.

Steps to be open to change

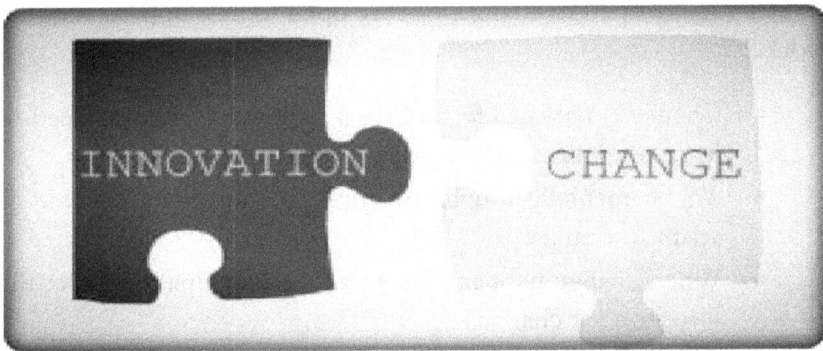

1. Realise you never have all of the information there is to have. You can always learn more.
2. Open your mind to new information, ideas, and opinions rather than instantly rejecting them.

3. If someone presents new information to you or their opinion, listen to what they're saying rather than arguing or batting them down.
4. Be honest with yourself about why you are upset or angry about the change, information, or opinion.
5. Don't be offended by other people's opinions and advice.
6. Analyse new ideas and information—assess the pros and cons for yourself.
7. Collect new information and experiences and use them to make creative solutions.
8. Use your mind as a tool to make changes.
9. See change as an opportunity, rather than fearing it.
10. Be brave and try new things—step out of your comfort zone.

So, open your mind to endless possibilities, to expansion, to new horizons. Opening your mind opens many paths that you thought were closed, and provides so many opportunities for success because you are not limiting yourself anymore.

Reminder

When you are open to change, you are open to new opportunities in your life:

- Change is part of life, and it's a part of life that we need to learn to embrace, rather than fighting or avoiding it.
- To be mentally tough, you need to be open and able to adapt to change.
- When change happens, be an active participant and set the direction for change.
- Recognise the opportunities present in change, rather than seeing the negatives.
- When you are open to change, you choose your reaction to it and the outcome, rather than letting life happen to you.

CHAPTER 9

Openness To Criticism
And Developing 24/7

"Criticism may not be agreeable, but it is necessary. It fulfils the same function as pain in the human body. It calls attention to an unhealthy state of things." -
Winston Churchill

In the last chapter, we looked at the importance of being open to change, new ideas, and new information. But it's also important to be open to criticism of ourselves. As humans, we tend not to take criticism well. But if you want to be mentally tough, you need to be able to take criticism and turn it into personal improvement.

Being open to criticism and developing 24/7 is an important part of mental toughness. This is because being open to criticism is an inherent part of self-improvement. Mental toughness involves a permanent attitude to self-improvement, so being open to developing 24/7 is crucial. If you're able to accept negative feedback about yourself or your work without reacting emotionally, you can improve yourself and do better in the future. So, in this chapter, you'll learn how to take criticism and be open to development.

What happens when we receive criticism?

Many people think they're open to criticism, but when it happens, they're actually not. When someone tells us something we don't like, we often get offended. You might feel hurt, upset, or angry. Instead of thinking about why they might say that, you don't consider that the person may be right. You get defensive, say something mean back to them, argue with them, or distance yourself. As a result, not being able to take criticism can lead to the end of friendships, relationships, or jobs.

For example, you ask your fiend whether it looks like you've lost any weight. They don't want to lie to you, so they say, "Not really, but you'll get there". You take great offence—obviously they think you're fat! How rude. How dare they say you haven't lost any weight. You're angry, and you decide to distance yourself from them. What you should do is wonder—why are they saying that?

Or at your appraisal, your boss tells you that you could take on more responsibility. You're hurt that they think you're not doing enough, and feel like they told you off. You don't want to hear that you could be doing more to improve, and you're offended that they think you should take on more—instead of seeing it as a compliment. What you should think is what am I doing that's causing them to say this? Sound familiar? Don't worry, you can learn to take criticism on board and use it to improve.

Unfortunately, most people don't appreciate any kind of feedback on themselves. In fact, people brag about having "a thick skin"—that is, actually *ignoring* criticism. Some people are renowned for being "sensitive"—being unable to hear criticism without falling apart. Responding defensively to criticism is usually a sign of low self-esteem, so if you find yourself doing this, you need to work on your self-confidence some more. True mental strength isn't batting off criticism, but taking it on board and learning something from it, then using it to improve.

Why we need to take criticism on board

Firstly, in a very basic sense, you can't go through life avoiding criticism. Throughout your life, you will have to deal with other people's opinions. Whether it's your boss, your coach, customer feedback, or friends giving you advice. Especially if you're doing something noticeable, like starting a new business, people will have plenty of feedback for you!

If you get upset or angry every time you get negative feedback, you'll expend a lot of your energy and waste a lot of time being emotional. You'll also be letting other people control your emotions. You won't be in control of the situation. You may also push people away or damage your relationship with them by reacting badly. If you say something offensive back, it might result in an argument and an end to the relationship. But if you take it well, your friendship will grow and strengthen because you can be honest with each other.

Importantly, other people's opinions and criticism will help you improve and develop. When you're working on your business, it's easy to lose sight of reality, and other people's opinions can provide this vital outside perspective. Whether it's spotting a fault with the process, a potential improvement, or a new method you can use. Criticism enables you to improve the process, object, or offering.

For example, if you're a CEO, a team member might point out that you've missed a gap in the process. As the CEO, you could take offence that they've pointed out your oversight—and think "How dare they speak to me like that, when I'm the CEO and they're just an employee?" But taking on board the feedback will help you improve the process. When you run a business, feedback is vital to its growth.

As an individual, criticism opens the way to vital self-development and personal growth. We live with ourselves every day, but it's often hard to see how we come across to others, so it's useful to get an outside perspective on ourselves. This might be a friend giving you a much-needed reality check, a stranger pointing out something you hadn't noticed before, or a colleague teaching you a new skill. Personal criticism enables you to develop new skills, qualities, and abilities.

Taking on board this criticism requires self-awareness and the understanding that you will make mistakes. So, if you're struggling to see the validity in somebody's criticism, you need to start being more honest with yourself, and do a self-appraisal. If you want to develop mental toughness, you need to be courageous enough to accept criticism.

How to take criticism well

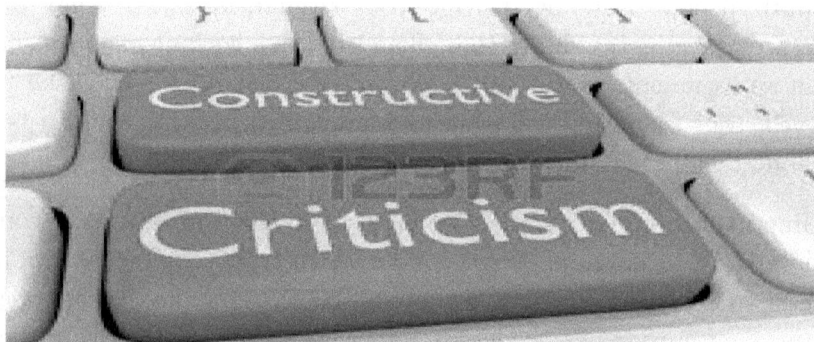

When somebody gives you negative feedback or criticism, follow this process:

1. Take a deep breath before you respond. This will stop the knee-jerk defensive reaction and enable you to control your emotions. **Respond, don't react**.
2. Think before you respond. Doing this means you won't say something that you'll regret later.
3. Be objective about *what* the person is saying, instead of being emotional about them having said it.
4. Remember that the person is most likely saying this to help you improve. Even if the person responding was rude or emotional, it will help you improve.

5. Be polite in your response to them. Thank them for the feedback and tell them you'll take it on board.

6. Remember that even if the feedback you received was hard to hear, it will help you to improve.

7. Instead of getting upset about the criticism, start by thinking how you can turn the criticism into an opportunity to improve.

Sometimes, the criticism you receive won't be useful because the person saying it was trying to put you down, having a bad day, or taking their anger out on you. When you're taking criticism on board, you need to learn which criticism is valuable and which is not. Often, you can spot the valuable criticism because it's clear and specific, or because you've heard it from several people, rather than just one angry person.

How to ask for feedback

When you realise how useful negative feedback is in helping you improve yourself or your business offering, you are likely to want more of it! However, it can be difficult to get useful, constructive feedback. To get good feedback:

1. Ask somebody to provide feedback on you or your business using words that demonstrate your openness to receiving it. Don't shout "What did I do wrong?!" Say calmly, "I'd like to find out where I could have done better..."

2. Start with open questions that enable you to hone in on the problem, such as "I'd like to find out your perspective" or "Do you have any recommendations on how I could improve?"

3. Then, move on to clear, precise, and specific questions, such as "What did you think about the end of the process?" This way, the feedback will be actionable and focused.

4. Ask the person to be honest, but when you ask them, be polite. That way, you will receive a response that is polite, rather than emotional.

5. Thank the person for their feedback, regardless of whether it was good or bad, polite or not. This will help them feel comfortable to provide feedback in the future.

If you're finding it difficult to speak to the person one-on-one, you could try a feedback survey or ask them to tell somebody they trust, who can then convey the message to you.

How to give feedback – CEOs and coaches

If you have to regularly provide feedback to players or staff, you need to learn to give helpful, constructive criticism if you want them to improve and not react badly. However, it can be just as difficult to give feedback as take it. Providing unhelpful feedback can cause their performance to deteriorate, and damage your relationship with them. It's important to note that high-performing staff are more likely to be open to feedback than low-performing staff.

To give useful feedback, you need to:

1. Do it in the right setting. Set up a one-to-one or appraisal, rather than saying it in the office in front of everyone.
2. Say it in the right tone. Don't shout at the person or speak emotionally—be objective.
3. Be honest but be kind. Don't sugar-coat the feedback, but don't be overly harsh.
4. Be specific and clear. Give them focused actions to work on in specific areas.
5. Ask them questions to help them understand and find solutions.
6. Ensure they understand what is being said to them by asking them to respond.

How to use feedback

So, now you know how to take criticism well. But the important thing is you need to use the information!

1. Stop. Don't just go back to what you were doing before and carry on as you were.
2. Think creatively how you can use the information to improve.
3. Set yourself practical, measurable goals to improve in this area.
4. Act on the information by making the change happen every day, consistently.
5. Measure your own performance to see whether you are improving.
6. Keep going despite difficulties.
7. Go back to the person who gave the feedback and share your progress.
8. Ask the person for more feedback to see whether other people can see the improvement.

For instance, if you're the CEO and you get feedback from a manager that the staff think you're unapproachable, set a goal to be more approachable within a month so staff feel they can come to you with ideas and feedback. Make changes, such as having an "open door policy" where staff can come in to speak to you, saying hi to your staff when you enter the office, asking staff to submit ideas to win a prize. Then ask your managers to get an update in monthly one-to-ones with staff.

Or if your coach tells you that your form is wrong when you're throwing the ball, set a goal to improve in two days. Start practising every day consistently. Watch videos of great players and how they throw. Read online tips and tutorials. Try different methods. Then ask your coach to re-evaluate your form at the end of a few weeks.

Embracing personal development

As you start to take feedback on board and turn it into improvements, you'll realise that development isn't a static thing. It's a 24/7 process. Developing and improving isn't about just doing it once and then being satisfied with your results. It's about continuously seeking feedback, and continuing to improve. There is always more knowledge out there, and you can always improve—using new methods, books, ideas, or research.

I've seen this in practise as a mental toughness expert. The people who truly develop mental toughness are those who embrace improvement as a lifestyle choice. Me included. I know that if I want to be the best expert, I need to continually improve myself. So I travel to expand my mind, read the latest articles and studies, study sports stars at the top of their game, and speak to mentally tough people and other experts doing the same role as me.

What all of the evidence says is **work on it every day**. Get better every day. The people who achieve success in the long term are the people who practise every day, who are always improving. Evidence shows that you need to keep practising every day to keep your mind active. Keep your skills sharp. In other words, use your skills or lose them.

Long-term development for sportspeople

Have you noticed that some players only win for a season, or a game, or a tournament? This is because from that win, they stop improving. They sit back on that win, while everyone around them keeps working hard to improve. They think that one-win means success, and they don't continue to improve every day. Or they don't realise that the field of sports changes every day, and they need to change with it.

On the other hand, the best players win over the long term—they're on the top of the pile for years. Not just because they're talented, but because they have mental toughness, because they embrace permanent development. American basketball player and coach Mike Krzyzewski said "I would take real toughness over talent any day. When you have both, then you have a true champion."

To keep improving, you need three key components:

Physical: Hard work—physically putting in all of your effort and looking after yourself.

Mental: Smart training—figuring out how to improve and allowing yourself to recover.

Emotional: Mental toughness—controlling your emotions and overcoming challenges.

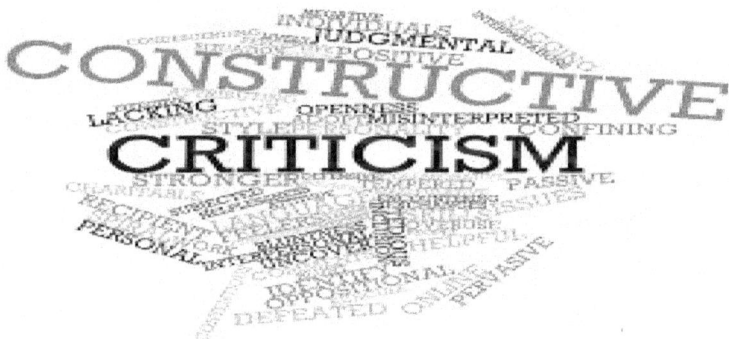

It's not enough to just have one of these components. If you just work hard but don't train smart, you'll overwork yourself and get burnt out. If you work hard and train smart but don't have mental strength, you'll fail when you reach critical challenges, and you won't get back up from them.

But if you work hard and train smart and have mental strength, you'll embrace challenges as opportunities to improve and you'll give your body time to recover. This is why athletes who have all three components have long careers instead of burning out after one season.

Reminder

You need to be prepared to receive feedback throughout your life. When you do,

- Take a deep breath and instead of reacting emotionally or defensively, think about what the person is saying and why they are saying it. Are they right?

- Take feedback as an opportunity to learn and improve yourself.
- Be open to criticism, as you can use it in your personal life, work, and in sports to improve your performance.
- Keep developing 24/7, every day—success happens over the long term.
- Invest in your long-term mental, emotional, and physical health.

CHAPTER 10

Turn Problems Into Opportunities

"Success is 99 percent failure" -Soichiro Honda

Everyone encounters problems and challenges in life. Some people persevere through them, while others let these problems stop them from achieving their goals. If you're mentally tough, you don't just persevere through your goals, but you actually turn them into opportunities for success and improvement.

Turning problems into opportunities is an important approach in mental toughness. This is because mental toughness means being committed to consistent daily action, and this doesn't stop when you encounter a problem. Mental toughness means seeing problems as opportunities, and turning each challenge into a possibility for improvement of yourself or your life.

So, in this chapter, we'll look at how to turn problems into opportunities for success. You'll see how to overcome problems and challenges and get back up when you're down. In the following chapter, we'll look at how to triumph over great adversity no matter what life throws at you.

Life is a lesson

Life becomes a lesson when the process of confronting problems and solving them is painful. In this process of solving problems lies the meaning of life. Problems require our courage and our wisdom to solve. Problems create our determination and our knowledge. Only because of problems do we grow mentally and spiritually. As Benjamin Franklin once said, "What hurts, teaches." Smart people learn from their mistakes and their problems—they carry their pain and they learn not to fear.

Unfortunately, most of us are not smart enough. Most of us fear pain, so we try to avoid problems. We set them aside for later, hoping they'll disappear. We try to ignore them, neglect them, pretend they don't exist. But if you want to be different tomorrow, then you have to do something different today. If today is just a consequence of yesterday, then tomorrow will simply be the result of today.

Most people don't see the full truth that life *is* difficult. It's supposed to be. Instead, they complain, more or less continuously, loudly or quietly, about their enormous problems, their burdens, and difficulties, as if life was supposed to be easy. Life is a chain of challenges. We're happy to moan about them, but do we want to solve them?

What happens when we encounter problems

In life, most of us fail to achieve our goals because when we encounter a problem along the way, we simply give up on our dreams. These problems can include challenges, obstacles, mistakes, failures, setbacks, frustrations, rejection, pain, and exhaustion. They can be mental, physical, or emotional. They can be as simple as having a bad day to being unable to beat your best time, pulling a muscle to making a mistake at work.

But when encounter these problems, we often quit our goals. We let these relatively minor problems stop us from achieving what we want to achieve. instead of accepting responsibility for giving up, we say that the circumstances have beaten us. We blame our lack of money, lack of time, or lack of resources. We blame other people's lack of faith in us. We'll literally look for anyone to blame except for looking in the mirror and taking responsibility for giving up on our dreams. This is because we expect the path to success to be easy.

Unfortunately, most people don't see what's involved in achieving extraordinary things. They admire athletes on TV who achieve amazing feats of strength or speed. They celebrate musicians who make music that brings joy, or authors who write incredible, inspiring books. What they don't see is the blood, sweat, and tears of the athlete, the rejections by music labels, or the pile of returned manuscripts on the doormat. They don't see the risk these extraordinary people made to achieve their dreams—the risk the took—the problems they overcame. If you want to succeed, you have to take the risk.

In reality, everyone encounters problems at some point in their life, particularly when they try to achieve their goals. The people who succeed in life aren't people who've never encountered problems—they're people who don't give up and don't let these problems stop them. You can be one of these people too.

How to overcome problems

What you need to realise is that when you're trying to develop a new skill, or achieve a goal, or reach your dreams, you *will* encounter problems. The path to success isn't smooth. You will inevitably face problems—you'll encounter pain, exhaustion, frustrations, setbacks, challenges, obstacles, and you'll make mistakes and sometimes fail. But you need to stay positive and focus on solutions instead of focusing on the problems and becoming a victim of circumstances.

But if you want to become good at something, succeed at something, you have to put in the effort and practice, practice, practice. Developing a new skill takes hours of work. So, when you say "I'm not good at writing" what you actually mean is "I haven't practised writing enough". I used to say that, and now I've written a book. There is no magic pill that will enable you to do—it takes hard work, practice, and effort. What it comes down to is that you have to put in the time, effort, and work to achieve your goals.

Despite encountering problems, you need to **keep going**. This is what mental toughness is about. It's about keeping going no matter what. You need to find a way through your problems, and the way through doesn't involve giving up. If you're struggling with this, think of it this way—if you give up, you're missing out on the reward for all of your hard work. If you keep going, you'll reap the rewards of your efforts and it will have been worth it. If you give up, then it wasn't worth it. Your time is limited, so don't waste it by giving up on something.

When you encounter a problem, remember...

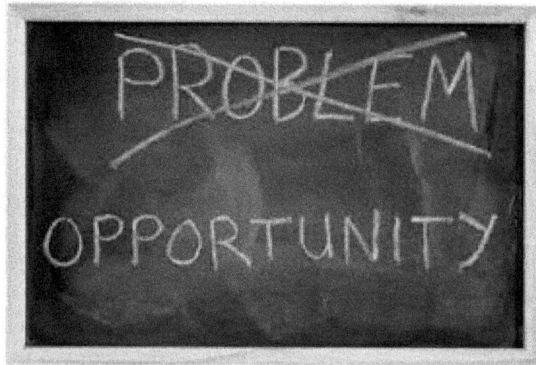

- Difficult times don't last forever—you just have to get through them.
- Problems are temporary—giving up is forever.
- You have greatness within you—show it.
- Don't run from challenges, face them head on.
- Make difficult decisions.
- Do the things you don't like doing.
- When you're knocked down, think about your goals and dreams...and get back up!
- What doesn't kill you makes you stronger.

- If you're having a bad time, hold your head up high.
- Reward yourself for small successes.
- Fight to protect your dreams.
- Quitting is not an option.

Turning problems into opportunities

When you start overcoming challenges, you become more able to overcome other challenges. You strengthen your mind, because you're telling it that you won't give up. When you overcome a challenge, you come out stronger and tougher than before. You develop mental toughness through these challenges—not through life being easy.

This is where turning problems into opportunities comes in. Problems are chances to become stronger, smarter, faster, more agile, better. If you don't encounter challenges, you won't test your own skills and abilities, and you won't improve. So, when you encounter a problem, see it as an opportunity to develop a new skill, gain more knowledge, do something better than before.

If you want to reach the heights of success, life won't be all picnics. If it is, then you're not aiming high enough. When life starts throwing difficulties your way, you're on your way to the top. The higher you want to get, the more difficult the challenges. This is about your mindset. You need to make the decision to see problems as opportunities.

Turning problems into opportunities requires perseverance. It's trying to exceed your limits, pushing through the pain, and fighting through lack of focus. It's about pushing your own limits—this is what mental toughness requires. It's not easy, and it's not supposed to be. If you avoid problems, or give up when you encounter them, you won't succeed. But if you put in the effort to fight through the problems, you'll achieve your goals.

Overcoming the situation

If you don't believe me, there are many famous examples of people overcoming problems through persistence. A great example is basketball legend Michael Jordan. Michael loved basketball as a kid, but was always losing to his brother. He was rejected for his high school basketball team. But he was determined to succeed. Every morning, he lifted weights and practised his skills. At the end of the summer, he was one of the best high school players and got a place at uni. He was drafted for the Chicago Bulls and became an NBA champion and MVP multiple times, as well as an Olympic gold medallist, and many more accolades.

Throughout this, he experienced failures, injuries, and loses. He knew how many times he'd missed a shot and how many games he'd lost. He failed numerous times, but always got back up again. He practised, practised, and practised some more. And he accounts his success to this mentality of never giving up. Despite encountering problems, he always got back up and kept trying.

How do I know about problems?

I know this because when I was young, my parents went to work every day, even when they were exhausted, even when they were ill. My dad worked in his shop, and my mum worked at the local hospital. It was tough back then to run your own business, post-communism, in Poland. But no matter what happened, my parents would say "When a situation knocks you down, get back up." As a child, I learned that this was mental toughness meant.

If you knock me down, I will get back up. Despite going through problems, my parents were first role models in life, and they taught me to be mentally tough. They didn't say "give up when it gets difficult". My mum sent me to learn English for a few years, and I knew she was paying for my lessons, so I didn't want to let her down. I wanted to learn English because I knew it would help me succeed in life, but I found it so difficult to learn—it's really nothing like Polish. I was determined to learn it.

The school was also tough—and the teachers purposely ensured we would fail. They didn't make us fail permanently, but enough to teach us mental toughness. If we failed a test or didn't do our homework, we did it until we got it right. One day, during an exam, I was really struggling. I was exhausted and couldn't focus. One of my teachers came over and said, "Are you going to give up or are you going to get up?" Suddenly, I was focused and I completed the exam.

The teacher was my second role model—she was tough, never gave up, never quit. Every time I got my English lessons, I said to myself "How tough are you?". I became determined to keep improving. Every day, I analysed what could I do better the next day. I was going to try harder and keep doing that every time. I saw my parents doing it. I was going to do it too.

After two years of lessons, I had my final exam. My parents were excited and believed that I would pass. I failed. I was the only one of twelve students who failed! I was devastated, I couldn't believe it, and cried to my mum that I let her down. She had worked hard to pay all the bills, to feed me, and pay for lessons, and I had failed. I lost faith in my ability, and I lost my confidence. I thought I would never be able to stand up on my own two feet and get a good job. Not being able to pass the English exam felt like a massive, insurmountable problem.

But after a few months, I decided to turn my failure into an opportunity for success. I applied for a work experience position in a hotel in Scotland. I didn't have to demonstrate my level of English or do any tests, I just needed industry experience. So, I told my parents I was going to Scotland, and in September 2004, I flew to Glasgow. I worked and lived in a small village near Helensburgh.

It was tough, as I didn't know nobody. I did nothing but work. I was an only child from a big city in a small place, from a different culture, and I was on my own, without being able to speak good English. What's more, it was hard to improve my English without having anyone to speak to. It could have defeated me, but I was determined to succeed. I could have just packed my bags and gone back to Poland, but I didn't.

In my head, I could hear my teacher's voice, "If you want to learn to speak English, go and learn it. If you want to be fluent in any language, go and prove it. Life isn't easy, but you never quit. Never. You may not have been the best, but you can always give your best". So, I turned the problem of having nothing to do into the opportunity to self-study on my days off, then I practised what I'd learned at work.

This combination helped me progress and learn English faster. My time in Scotland was tough, but it was worth it. Every day I practised, working hard to learn the language, and every day I improved, despite my difficult circumstances. Looking back, I realise that this was the real test for me, not the exam I had failed— because this test made me truly mentally tough. It made me not give up. I persisted, despite the problems, despite lack of confidence in my abilities, despite being on my own. I pushed past my own limits. I became confident. So, believe me when I say it's possible, because I've proved that it's possible.

As a parent, how do you help your children overcome problems?

As a parent, you might be wondering how to inspire your children to overcome problems, particularly if they need help in school or in their sport. The first thing you need to do is evaluate whether you are helping or hindering them, as we discussed earlier in the *What Is Mental Toughness?* chapter. I don't need to tell you that if you're hindering them—stop right now and start helping them.

Then, consider your role as being there to encourage them. For example, when I was younger, I wanted to learn to play basketball. I imagined playing like my hero at the time, Michael Jordan. My parents bought me a little basketball, and I joined local streetball teams. My parents said, "If you learn the basic skills, we will buy you a bigger, more professional basketball." I was more motivated and visualised a new basketball, the basketball the Michael Jordan played with it. My older friends from streetball teams taught me the basics, but I learned more as I was self-motivated. My parents saw this and bought me books so I could read and improve.

When I applied to join a junior local basketball team, my new coach said "I heard you can play a ball. If you are good you can join the team." I had a choice and vision. My coach asked me whether I could play point guard. I said I couldn't. I tried, and I couldn't play this challenging position. I couldn't pass the ball to an open player at the right time, dribble under pressure, or shoot well with a defender close to me. I felt useless and I wanted to quit!

So, my parents asked my auntie to speak to me. She was also a basketball player, and she said to me "If you ever get overwhelmed, break it down. Practise one part, then add the second and third parts. Put them together and you will learn." So, I practised for hours and hours for a few months and learned the position, even better than my coach! My coach asked me how I did it. So, I showed him and taught him! The lesson here is that we can always learn from each other. As a parent, you need to have the humility to let your children teach you too. You could even suggest that you can work together to improve, such as learning a new language together.

As a coach, how do you help players to overcome problems?

As a coach, you might wonder how to help players overcome difficult times. As a coach, I used the lessons I learned as child to help my players overcome hurdles. Whether it was struggling to adapt to a new position, overcoming an injury, having a bad day on the court, or having home life problems that affected their playing. I encouraged them to put in the effort and hard work needed to succeed when they encountered injuries or dips in performance—to be persistent and stay focused.

I also taught them to forget mistakes and keep going until they succeeded, to focus on each play as it happened and not on errors they'd just made. This way, they had less "bad days" as they didn't compound one bad play into a bad game by giving themselves a hard time and losing focus.

Sometimes, players were struggling to improve and getting frustrated with themselves because they felt they were stuck at a certain level and were limited to staying there. I taught them that they can overcome any hurdle when they are having the self-confidence that they can do it. Much of overcoming problems in sports is believing you can get better, jump that hurdle, and beat that time or previous score. Like Michael Jordan says, "limits like fears are often just an illusion."

Other times, players were struggling because they saw a problem and believed they were trying to overcome it, but in reality, they were just complaining and not actually doing anything. When this was the case, I sat them down and made them look in the mirror. I made them have an honest conversation with themselves about whether they were really putting in the effort to overcome the problem.

Sometimes, players saw problems because they didn't get along with other teammates, and it was causing tension. When this happened, I talked to them about self-confidence and the importance of everyone playing as a team, respecting each other, and working together.

I also considered my role as the coach and how I was communicating with them and working with them to improve. I realised I sometimes reacted with emotion to players, such as yelling when they made a mistake, instead of responding objectively. This didn't bring out the best performance in them. So now I respond rather than reacting emotionally. I take a deep breath and focus myself.

In other words, I taught my players the importance of mental toughness to overcome problems.

As the CEO, how do you help staff overcome problems?

As the manager, you will offer encounter staff struggling with problems in the office. Often, the answers are the same as if you're coaching a team. But sometimes, the problems occur because staff don't understand their place in the company or the aims of the company. If you have lots of staff who seem to be having problems, it could be that the communication they're getting isn't good enough.

Perhaps they don't understand the vision of the company so are struggling to act in a way that helps the company move in the right direction. Perhaps they have heard rumours the company is making a loss and people might be made redundant and so they are worried about losing their job rather than focusing on work. Perhaps they've heard you complaining about other staff members and they don't trust your integrity or have any confidence as you.

Be honest with yourself whether you are communicating openly and honestly with your staff. For example, if the company is going through a restructure, do your staff know this is happening before the local press report potential redundancies? Do your staff understand the process of restructure and whether their job is safe? Do they know what is required of them in the new structure?

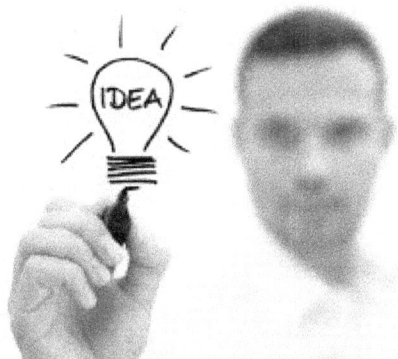

If you communicate well, and in a timely manner, staff will be able to adapt to change and overcome problems better than if they find out last minute, from outside sources, or overhear it at the water cooler. Staff need to understand why they are doing things, what the company's aims are, and how they fit in with that.

Reminder

- Help other people overcome problems by considering whether you are part of the problem and encouraging the person to develop mental toughness.
- Realise that life isn't supposed to be easy and you will inevitably face challenges in life. Don't try to avoid challenges or problems, or hide from them.
- The bigger your aims in life, the more difficult the challenges will be.
- When you do encounter problems—stay positive and focus on solutions, not the problems.
- Persevere when you encounter problems—push through the pain, push your own limits.
- When you encounter a problem, see it as an opportunity to develop a new skill, gain more knowledge, and do something better than before.
- See problems as a chance to become better, stronger, smarter, faster, and more agile.
- Overcoming your problems is the path to success.

CHAPTER 11

How To Win Against Adversity

"Success is to be measured not so much by the position that one has reached in life as by the obstacles which he has overcome" - Booker T. Washington

In the previous chapter, we looked at turning short-term or smaller problems into opportunities to improve. Now you know how to overcome a bad day or a short illness, and how to help others overcome them. But what about when it's a particularly traumatic situation? Or when we continue to face big problems in life? How do we fare when we encounter *true adversity*?

Often, we let it defeat us. But if you want to achieve lasting change in life, you need to learn to triumph over adversity. Doing so is a major part of mental toughness, because adversity is part of life. Winning against adversity actually helps us develop mental toughness, because each adverse situation we overcome makes us stronger. So, in this chapter, we'll look at how to win against adversity.

What does it mean to "win against adversity"?

You often hear the phrase "triumph over adversity" or similar, but what does it actually mean? Well, unlike small challenges that we need to overcome to achieve a goal, winning against adversity means succeeding when everything is going against you. It means overcoming great difficulties and **beating the odds**. It can be anything from having a difficult start in life to having a disability or a long-term debilitating illness, or experiencing the loss of a job or family member. It can be experiencing a succession of smaller problems over a long period of time.

When we encounter adversity, we often let it beat us in life. Sometimes, we develop a victim mentality and start to think that life is unfair to us. We blame our lack of success on life being unfair, and convince ourselves that other people succeed because they have better circumstances, more money, more luck, and less problems than us. We say things like "life has dealt me a tough hand" and "other people have it easier than me". We use adversity as an excuse for giving up on ourselves.

Sometimes, it may seem like everyone has an easier life than you. Maybe you got a bad start in life and had a difficult childhood. Maybe you suffered serious health problems or lost loved ones. But this is not a reason to give up. Some of the best athletes and businesspeople in the world experienced great adversity and overcame it. In fact, these traumatic experiences are sometimes the very thing that inspired them to succeed. Winning against adversity means succeeding no matter what life throws at you and regardless of how difficult it seems.

How to overcome adversity

First, you need to accept that adversity is part of life. As Havelock Ellis wrote, "Pain and death are part of life. To reject them is to reject life itself." When you accept this, you'll spend less time being frustrated that things are so difficult to you, thinking that life is unfair to you, comparing yourself to others, or complaining about your situation. Bad things will always happen in life.

Second, you need to realise that experiencing adversity actually helps you reflect, understand yourself better, enhance your relationships with others, and make you humble. In fact, every adverse situation you've encountered in life has made you who you are. In other words, remember "what doesn't kill you makes you stronger". Experiencing and overcoming adversity makes you stronger as a person.

Third, you need to realise this, we all do well for ourselves when things are going well in our lives. But that's not true toughness. That's not mental strength. What distinguishes the great people, the winners, is how they triumph during the difficult times.

Strategies to win against adversity

Increase your expectations

One strategy to win against adversity applies particularly if you've experienced a tough start in life. Perhaps you had no money, or were told to accept your lot, or were beaten down or bullied by someone. When we encounter these situations, we start to think that we don't deserve anything more than what we have. We accept that as our lot in life, and we have low expectations of ourselves and what we can achieve. We think we have to just accept our circumstances, and our unfortunate circumstances begin to define us.

If we grow up in poverty, we think we're doomed to live that way forever, that there's no chance of earning a six-figure income. We define ourselves as "the poor man" and we don't strive for anything bigger. But you can change that—you just have to dream bigger and increase your expectations.

Step 1: Make your goals a priority. In life, we often have a list of things we **want** to do and things we **must** do. The "must" list tends to include basic survival tasks, such as eating, sleeping, and going to work. The "want" list includes improvement tasks, such as learning to speak another language, becoming the best at our chosen sport, or opening our own business. Our goals are on the "want" list, but if we move them to the "must" list, we become more serious about making them happen. We will find a way, like we'd find food if we were starving.

Step 2: Next, your goals must be consistent with your self-beliefs. If you have a goal but don't believe you can achieve it, you won't achieve it. You have to believe you can overcome your situation. This goes back to having self-confidence as we discussed earlier. Often, we think we can't achieve our goals because our self-beliefs are limited and negative. When you think you can't do something, look at where that "can't" comes from. It comes from inside ourselves, either because someone has told us we can't or because we've told ourselves we can't. But we can do it—remove those limitations.

Step 3: Change your self-identity. We adapt ourselves to become the person we have defined ourselves as, or the person other people have defined us as. For example, if society has defined us as "poor", we accept we're poor and live that life. If we have defined ourselves as "a failure", we become that failure. So, you need to change the definition of your self-identity to be someone better.

Step 4: Increase your expectations. If your only expectations in life are to live on the breadline, to scrape by every month, to pay the bills and survive, then that's all you'll achieve. If your expectations are to work 9-5, that's all you'll achieve. Increase your expectations in life—to earn six figures, to own your own business, or whatever big dream you want.

Step 5: Find the motivation. When we've changed our identity and self-beliefs, we need the motivation and energy to make the change happen. Often, this comes from having a clear reason why we want to achieve it. For example, if we decide we simply want to be filthy rich but with no reason, we won't achieve it. Knowing the specific reason helps us plan to make it happen.

Tips on how to win against adversity

When you're going through a difficult time, these tips will help:

- Realise that you are stronger than you think.

- Realise that you deserve to be happy and to achieve great things in life.
- Make an effort to smile and hold yourself tall.
- Approach the situation with a positive attitude.
- Remember that you're not the only person experiencing adversity. Most people experience adversity during their lives, and they make it through. You can make it through too.
- Don't see adversity as something bad, but something that will help you to become stronger, better, smarter, faster, or more resilient.
- Control what you can control and stop worrying about what you can't control.
- Find a way to succeed in the situation—think creatively. There's always another way.
- Don't see failures or mistakes as bad things. See them as learning experiences.
- If you're struggling to find inspiration to overcome the adversity, think of a loved one who means everything to you and be inspired by them to overcome the situation. If you have children, be an inspiration to them and show them you win against adversity.
- Find a mentor (a colleague, teacher, friend, or family member) who you trust. They can help you during difficult times. You can pay it back during their difficult times.
- Write down all of things in life that you have to be thankful for.
- Remember every time you have overcome difficult circumstances in the past.
- Write down your aims, goals, and dreams in life and put them somewhere prominent so you see them often and are inspired by them, such as on the fridge or as your phone screen.

- Realise that the end goal, dream, or new life will be worth the effort and pain.
- Read motivational quotes or books. Watch inspirational videos or people.

What happens when you make excuses

Often, people are unhappy with their lives or a situation in their lives, but they make excuses for why they're not doing something about it or blame other people or circumstances for their lack of success. This can be for many reasons, such as:

- Fear of change, leaving their comfort zone
- Fear of ridicule from others or disapproval
- Fear of being disappointed if they don't achieve it
- Fear of failure
- Fear of taking responsibility
- Lack of self-confidence and negative self-beliefs

In this situation, the easiest way to overcome adversity is stop talking about it, complaining about it, thinking about it, worrying about it, planning for it, making excuses for it, and **just start doing it**. The only way to make change happen is with **action**. Complaining about your situation won't change it. Planning won't make it better. Remember that developing mental toughness means putting in consistent effort every single day. There is a reason sports giant Nike have the slogan "Just Do It".

You might think that making excuses for not making changes is easier than trying to make changes. It might seem easier in the short term as you're not putting in any work, but it's not easier in the long term. In the long term, making excuses will make your life harder, because you won't have achieved your goals, improved your life, or made life any easier for yourself. You'll feel stressed and unhappy for longer because you haven't changed your circumstances.

What's more, people make a decision about you and whether they want to be around you based on how you react to adversity. Making excuses will eventually push away friends or family who are fed up with your complaining. It will prevent you from getting promotions at work or gaining big business opportunities, because nobody wants to deal with someone who makes excuses. You'll miss out on opportunities. Making excuses will stop you from reaching your full potential. However, it's never too late to make a change, to improve your life, or to banish bad habits.

How to banish excuses forever

- If you're scared of change, focus on the benefits you'll gain from the new situation and how much better life will be.
- If you're worried what others will think, think of the positive change they will see in you when you start making changes, making your life better, and achieving your dreams. If they criticise you, take the criticism and use it to improve.
- If you're worried about failing or being disappointed, remember that failure is a normal part of life and you can learn from it and use it to become stronger in the future.
- If you're scared of taking responsibility, realise that only you are in control of your life and nobody can change it for you. You are responsible for your own life.
- If you have a lack of self-confidence, start making small changes to build your confidence. If you have negative self-beliefs, work on improving your beliefs and seeing the good in yourself.

Follow this process:

1. **Be honest with yourself.** Often, we don't realise we're making excuses. So when you find yourself saying "I can't" or "it's not possible" etc, think about what you're saying and why. Is it really not possible? Can you really not do it? Most of the time, you'll realise you're making an excuse.

2. **Reword yourself.** Instead of saying "I can't", change it to "I can". Instead of saying "it's not possible", change it to "it is possible".

3. **Remember you only live once.** Don't waste your time being unhappy with your situation and making excuses for not making changes. Channel your excuses into creative solutions instead, so rather than thinking of excuses, think of ways to succeed.

4. **Take responsibility.** Realise that only you control your life and only you can make it better.

5. **Click "reset".** Realise that this is an opportunity to stop making excuses and start making your life better. It doesn't matter how old you are or what situation you're in. There's always time to make a change.

6. **Start making it happen.** Set some goals, make a plan of how you will start achieving them with small daily actions, then start making the change happen with consistent efforts every day. At the end of every day, check in with yourself to see whether you made it happen.

Overcoming adversity for sportspeople

Many sportspeople get distracted or affected by the aspects of their game that they don't have control over, such as referees or umpires, the other players, equipment, the crowd, the weather, or the environment. In this situation, the most important way to overcome adverse situations is control what you can control. Adverse conditions are a major part of sports, so you need to learn to deal with them.

- You can't control the environment, but you can control how you react to it and plan for it.
- Make sure you've fully prepared yourself, as that is within your control.
- Make the best possible circumstances for yourself—from smart training to good nutrition and sufficient rest.

- If you're worried about the conditions, go to the venue in advance and check it out.
- Make a plan for changing circumstances so you're not caught off guard in adverse circumstances. Remember that everyone competing is up against the same conditions as you.

If you think back over all of your losses, consider whether the loss was a reason within your control or outside your control. If you're being honest with yourself, the majority were within your control. They weren't a result of the conditions or external factors, but within your mind. You need to control your mind to push through these adverse conditions—control your anxiety, confidence, and concentration.

To achieve long-term success, you need to put in consistent effort every single day. You need to push harder, and aim higher, even when your competitors would have given up because they faced adversity. You need to learn from difficult experiences and come back even stronger. You need to be dedicated and disciplined to achieve long-term success despite facing difficult circumstances. If you encounter adversity and this makes you give up on your goals, you won't achieve success.

When you look at the top sportspeople, they are extremely self-motivated to overcome adversity. As a result, they triumph over adverse situations that are common in high-level or elite sports, such as injury, illness, burnout, exhaustion, going stale, and losing to opponents. They have clear life goals, and this gives them a strong sense of direction—so when they encounter rough tides, they're committed to reaching their destination and aren't swayed from their course. They also have self-confidence and believe that they can achieve their goals, which motivates and encourages them.

When you're struggling with adverse situations, it's tempting to think that top sports stars must have lived an easy life and never encountered the kind of difficult situation you may be experiencing. However, there are many sports heroes who overcome extremely adverse conditions and risen to the top of their chosen sport. Consider star footballer Cristiano Ronaldo.

He was raised in poverty, got diagnosed with a heart condition at 14 that meant he would have to stop playing football, but had the operation and then went back to training a few days later. His dad died of alcoholism when Cristiano was 20, but he kept going in pursuit of his dreams. His goal was to become one of the world's best players within three years when he was given the prized no. 7 jersey at Manchester United. With persistence, he became one of the best players of our time despite growing up with adversity. Now, he gives a large amount of his wealth charity to help other people overcome their circumstances.

Overcoming bullying

There's a misconception that only weak people can be bullied. But anyone can be bullied, whether it's at work, home, school, or online. Bullying has various forms, including physical violence, mental abuse, name-calling, cyberbullying, sexual abuse, threatening, or teasing. However, developing mental toughness will help you deal with and overcome bullying.

When you're experiencing bullying, either at school or at work or somewhere else, it can be difficult to focus on your goals. What's more, it can seriously affect your confidence and mental health, and even cause you to quit your job, avoid school or work, and not want to leave the house. It can affect your trust in relationships, and have long-lasting effects if you don't overcome it.

I know how unpleasant bullying can be because a few years ago, my wife was bullied at work by her boss. She worked in small, very busy café and the manager there used to shout at her and the other staff. He told them they were too slow and not good enough, and he banned them from talking to each other. My wife was very upset and stressed out about this, and this didn't help the situation because she started making mistakes. This made him shout even more. Eventually, my wife decided it was best to leave the job.

However, bullying can be overcome, and this is how…

1: Identify the reason it's happening.

Firstly, identify why you are being bullied. What is it that the bully is picking on? Why do they dislike you? Sometimes it's just because you're different—you look different, dress different, listen to different music, or say different things. If this is the case, remember that everyone is unique and there is nothing wrong with being different. Be yourself and be proud of who you are.

Sometimes the reason relates to the bully themselves, such as their own lack of self-esteem. For example, when my wife left her job, she discovered that her manager was actually addicted to drugs. If this is the case, realise that the bullying is nothing to do with you.

2: Tell someone what's going on

It's vital to tell someone what's happening, as they can help you resolve the situation and provide support. This may be a teacher, counsellor, friend, or family member—someone you trust. They'll keep the information confidential and will be able to help you. Your friends and family will support you through it.

3: Stand up to the bully

When you know why it's happening and have told someone, prepare yourself to stand up to the bully. When you do this, stand tall, speak confidently, and make eye contact with them. Tell them in no uncertain terms that you will not be picked on, that you are happy with who you are, and to leave you alone.

4: Ignore them

When you've stood up to the bully, any other time you see them, just ignore them. Don't look at them, pretend they're not there, and surround yourself with a support group.

Overcoming emotional pain

If there's one thing that's certain in life, it's that we will all encounter pain at some point. Whether it's physical pain or mental pain, we need to be able to deal with and overcome it. Often, we can deal with physical pain by taking medicine or improving our physical health, and we're usually comfortable telling other people about our physical pain.

But when it comes to emotional or mental pain, we often don't know how to overcome it, and we feel uncomfortable telling others what we are experiencing, even though we all experience mental pain during our lives. For example, we all experience the loss of a loved one, whether it's a parent or friend passing away, or even the end of a close relationship.

Pain due to loss is one of the most difficult types of pain to overcome, but it is possible. First, you need to understand your feelings and realise they are normal. There are various theories on humans' reactions to loss, but the emotions we experience often include shock, denial, anger, depression, sadness, anxiety, and helplessness.

This can involve feeling angry at your loved one for lying and leaving you alone. You can feel detached from your surroundings, or blame yourself for the person's death or leaving. The important thing to realise is that these emotions are normal.

Secondly, you shouldn't try to stop yourself from feeling sad. You need to allow yourself time to grieve. You need to realise that overcoming emotional pain isn't immediate—it's not like taking a paracetamol and waiting 20 minutes. Getting over emotional pain can take between a year and 18 months, but it will get better with time.

One way to help overcome the pain is to retain your daily routine and consistent daily actions. This will also be helped by eating healthily, exercising regularly, and getting sufficient sleep and rest time. While it may be tempting to drink alcohol or drugs, avoid these influences as they will not help in the long run or when the effects of the alcohol have worn off.

Thirdly, you need to ensure you talk to people. While you may not feel like talking, it can really ease your pain to tell someone how you're feeling. Whether you speak to a friend or family member, a counsellor or healthcare professional, you will gain help and support. You might not feel ready for counselling at the beginning, but over time it might feel right for you.

By allowing yourself time to grieve, talking openly with others, and ensuring you maintain positive daily actions, you will overcome the pain in time.

Affirmations to overcome emotional pain

To overcome emotional pain, I use affirmations. Here are some of the ones I use and an explanation of why they are true —they might help you:

1. **Everything arises and passes.** If you can just learn to be still and handle whatever is happening, it will pass. Every time.

2. **Nothing happens without a reason.** Setbacks and obstacles exist for a reason. They are meant to be there. They are there to see who wants it most. *How bad do you want it?* When you encounter an obstacle, take the mess and turn it into the message. Take the test and make it a testimony. Obstacles are there to see how we respond. Ask any successful person and they will tell you that obstacles are there to be turned into opportunities.

3. **I don't need to know why this is happening right now. I just need to deal with it.** You almost never understand why something is happening while it's happening. Later, when you've come out the other side, it will become visible, and you'll have the chance to gain perspective and see whether changes need to be made.

145

4. **It's all perfect the way it is.** This can be a tough one to swallow, but if you can embrace this idea, then you're well on the way to a happier life. Everything about you and your life today is the culmination of everything that's ever happened—how could it possibly be any other way?

Importantly, this is not about trying to change how you feel at the moment, as you can't force yourself to feel better. It's about planting seeds and giving your mind the chance to step back from itself.

Reminder

To win against adversity, you need to embrace the following approach:

- Accept that adversity is part of life and instead of seeing it as something bad, realise that it actually helps you become a stronger person and develop mental toughness.
- Remember "what doesn't kill you makes you stronger".
- Banish excuses for why your life isn't what you want it to be—stop complaining about adverse situations and start making positive change happen.
- The only way to make change happen is with **consistent action.**
- Start making small actions every day to overcome your circumstances, as this will build your self-confidence and help you see that you can make changes, beat the odds, improve your situation, and triumph against adversity.
- Increase your expectations for yourself and your life.
- Be persistent, positive, open to new ideas, opportunities, and opinions.
- Think creatively to find a way to succeed in any adverse situation.

CHAPTER 12

Work On Your Body

"Health is a relationship between you and your body." - Terri Guillemets

We've talked a lot in this book about working on your mind. But it's also important that you work on your body. After all, your mind and body are connected and heavily influence each other. To give yourself the best possible chance of succeeding, achieving your goals, and developing mental toughness, you need to ensure your body is in top form too.

Working on your body is actually a really important part of mental toughness. This might sound strange, since mental toughness is in the mind, but as you've learned, mental toughness is developed through physical action. This means that if you're not physically healthy or fit, it's more difficult to maintain the consistent daily physical action needed for mental toughness.

What's more, looking after your body means you'll live longer and experience less health problems, both physical and mental. Thus, means you'll enjoy life more and be more able to achieve your goals. So, in this final chapter, you'll see how to create the best conditions for your body.

The benefits of exercise

No surprises here—one of the vital things you need to do (if you don't already) is exercise. Lots of people don't enjoy exercise, feel like they don't have time, and make excuses. But exercise is so important in keeping you healthy, both in body and mind. Exercising reduces your risk of diseases by a staggering 50% and help you to live a longer life, up to 30% longer. It can reduce your risk of:

- Cancer
- Stroke
- Diabetes
- Heart disease
- Stress
- Depression
- Dementia
- Alzheimer's
- Erectile dysfunction

Physically, it improves your weight, strength, posture, flexibility, mental strength, and stamina. The increased circulation also improves your health and helping you feel better. Exercise also increases the quality of your life and mental health, and is actually known to have a similar effect to anti-depressants, only without taking medication. It can improve your mood and energy levels, help you sleep better, and release stress and tension. It also helps you become more social and feel happier with your health and appearance, so it improves your self-esteem.

The trouble is, our lives are very sedentary these days, as many of us work office jobs where we sit down for long hours, and increases in technology means we do less hard, manual work. Computers wash our clothes, dishes, and cars. We can order our shopping from the internet and have someone deliver it. We drive to work or sit on public transport. We spend hours sat down watching TV or surfing the net. Studies suggest that most people spend more than 6 hours sat down every day. What's more, the food we eat is often processed. This lifestyle isn't good for our health, so we need to find a way to incorporate exercise into our daily lives.

How do I start?

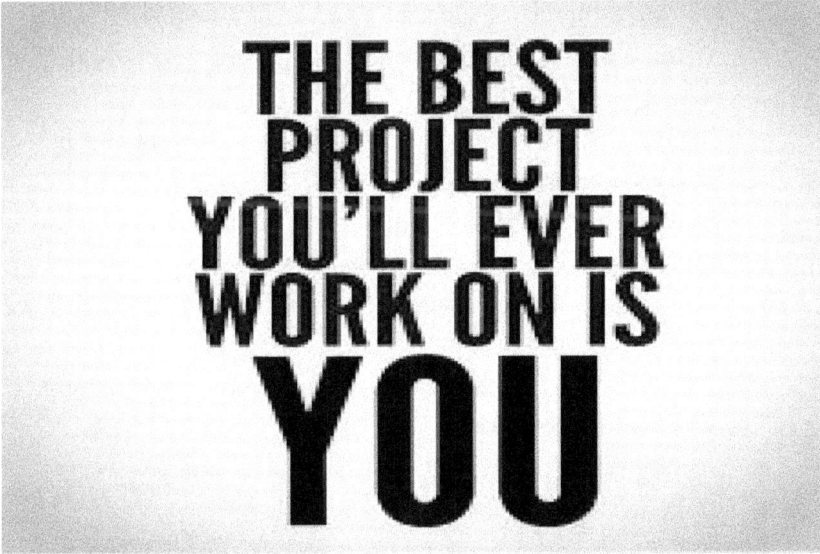

THE BEST PROJECT YOU'LL EVER WORK ON IS YOU

If you've never really exercised before, it can be hard to know where to start. But, it's easier than you expect to get started, and there's always something you can do even if you aren't used to exercise or are limited in time and finances. You just need to start small with daily actions and work your way up.

Whether you can't afford to join the gym, don't currently have much spare time, or are new to exercise, there's always a fitness plan that will suit your circumstances. If you can't afford a gym membership or classes, try free online videos and use your resources at home. If you don't have much time, combine exercise with your normal weekly activities. If you have health problems, ask your doctor what exercise would help. If you don't know where to start, have a personal training session and the trainer will help you develop a plan to suit your fitness level. Don't make excuses for yourself—exercise is free and you can get started at home.

So, try these ideas:

- Switch your daily drive or commute to work or shopping with walking or cycling. To start small, get off a stop early and walk the rest of the way.
- At the weekend, get involved with playing sports with your kids.
- Put on your favourite music and dance around the house, working up a sweat.
- Watch exercise videos online or on TV and practise at home.
- Join a local dance or exercise class where the instructor will check you're doing it right.
- Go swimming regularly, especially if you have asthma or lung health problems.
- Make it social by inviting your friends or family.
- Walk up the stairs instead of taking the lift.
- Instead of getting a coffee with your friends, go for a walk and talk.
- Get out in the garden and mow the lawn, plant plants, and breathe in the natural air.
- Stand up and walk around when you're on the phone.
- Exercise in the morning before work, or after work.
- Make better choices with your diet, such as switching an unhealthy piece of food for a healthy one every day.
- Remember, small consistent daily actions are best.

You only need to start small at first—so you could walk for 10 minutes three times a week. Then aim for half an hour three times a week. Eventually, aim for 150 minutes of moderate exercise, such as 10 minutes twice a day every day of the week, or whatever breakdown of the 150 minutes suits you.

Moderate means working up a sweat and increasing your heart rate. This can be high-intensity running, low-intensity yoga, or something different. The great thing is you'll start noticing a change straight away. Once you've eased yourself and your body into exercise, then work your way up to 3 hours every week.

Start doing this for a week and write down how you feel at the beginning of the week. Then write down how you feel at end of each workout and at the end of the week. By the end of the week, you should see that your mental strength has started to improve and you start to feel better mentally. As you start to see your improvement, you will develop self-confidence and mental toughness.

Tips when exercising

- Remember to always warm up before you exercise (such as stretching) and cool down afterward (such as gentle walking).
- Don't overexert or overextend yourself. Be self-aware and pay attention to what your body is telling you to avoid injury or illness.
- Check that the exercises are appropriate for your age and level of fitness.
- Check you're doing the exercises right by asking a personal trainer to show you the correct form and check your form.

What if I have a medical condition?

If you have a medical condition that makes it difficult to work out, it can be hard to know whether a particular type of exercise is possible for you and will be good for your health. The important thing to remember is that there's always something you can do to improve your health—you just need to pick something suitable and appropriate for your condition, lifestyle, and level of fitness.

The first thing to do is speak to your doctor to check what exercise or activity they recommend and to ensure that you won't damage your health further. For example, if you're asthmatic, your doctor may suggest swimming or yoga, rather than high-intensity running or spin classes. They might even be able to recommend local exercise classes. Exercises that might be suitable are:

- Low-impact exercises and stretches
- Walking
- Water aerobics or swimming
- Yoga or tai chi
- Gardening
- Dancing

Then you can work with a personal trainer who is aware of your condition and they will help ensure your fitness plan suits your health profile.

If you're older and are concerned about injuring your joints, try to avoid weight-bearing exercises such as running or aerobics. You can take up low-impact exercises such as tai chi or gardening.

What if I'm struggling to find the time?

One of the main reasons people don't engage in regular exercise is a lack of time, whether it's because your job is intense, you have other commitments, or have a family to look after. However, your health is vital, so you need to make time for looking after yourself.

To make the time, you first need to know where you're spending your time. Keep a diary for a few weeks and then identify things you could remove from your life to make time for exercise. You may need to go back to the chapter on saying "no". Cut out the time-wasting activities such as checking social media all the time. Save time by ordering your shopping online rather than going out to the supermarket. At work, outsource nonessential tasks to a freelancer or delegate them to a team member.

Then find timeslots to exercise based on the 150-minute ideal. This may be half an hour five times a week or 20 minutes every day.

Finding these timeslots may require some creative thinking, and may mean combining or replacing daily activities. For example, you could walk to work instead of taking the bus. You could park further away from the office. You could switch the lift for the stairs.

How do I stay motivated?

One of the hardest parts of exercise is staying motivated, particularly if you don't enjoy it. But remember, you need to keep going until it becomes a habit. To stay motivated, try the following:

- Choose the exercises or activities that you enjoy the most
- Ask a friend or family member to be your workout buddy
- Join a group exercise class or running club
- Ask your loved ones to support your efforts
- Set achievable and realistic short-term goals to improve your health
- You can set bigger goals in the long term
- Reward yourself for committing to exercise, but not with unhealthy snacks

Nutrition that helps with mental toughness

To develop mental toughness, your body needs to be healthy. Part of this involves eating well, not just exercising. Some people try specific diets to improve their health, but often these involve cutting out certain food groups. All food groups are fine in moderation unless you are allergic to a food or food group. If you believe you are allergic to a food group, such as wheat, please consult your doctor before removing it from your diet.

In general, a balanced diet is the best kind for your body, where you eat each food group in moderation and limit your intake of food, drink, and consuming things that are bad for your health. It's widely known that certain items are bad for your health, so try to reduce or avoid:

- Alcohol

- Cigarettes
- Fizzy/carbonated drinks
- Processed food
- High-fat or processed meat
- Fast food

Good foods to eat:

- Nuts, oats, and seeds
- Fruits such as blackberries, blueberries, tomatoes, oranges, strawberries, kiwis, and bananas
- Very dark chocolate
- Oily fish such as salmon and sardines
- Leafy green vegetables such as broccoli, spinach, kale, and cabbage
- Other veg such as beetroot, asparagus, potatoes, and celery
- Garlic
- Eggs
- Lentils

If you don't like some of these good foods right now, try the exercise mentioned earlier of replacing bad foods with good ones and developing mental toughness by eating things you don't like.

Mental toughness and the body

When it comes to mental toughness, you might think you will see the change happen physically. But it's important to realise that mental toughness isn't visible. It's not something you will see in your body shape, athleticism, physical abilities, or bodily strength. That doesn't mean you won't be able to sense or feel it, or know it's there. Mental strength is an attitude, a way of life, a way of being.

Reminder

Your physical health is vital to your mental health and to achieving your goals. If your body isn't well, then your mind will be less able to focus and you'll fall into negative thinking and will lack self-confidence. To look after your health, you need to:

- Exercise every day or several times a week (aiming for 150 minutes of exercise per week).
- Have a balanced diet.
- See a doctor if you have health conditions before deciding which exercise to take up.
- Start small and work your way up to bigger fitness goals.
- Get proper rest/relaxation time (such as meditation) and a good amount of sleep (ideally 7.5-8 hours per night).
- Ensure you make the time to look after your health.
- Avoid anxiety and negative stressors.

FINAL THOUGHTS

For many years, I have analysed why some people can achieve whatever they want while others can't. Take the NBA (National Basketball Association) as an example. It's the best basketball league in the world in terms of organisation, finance, and level of sport. Every player who plays in this league is a remarkable person. The level of physicality of all the players in this league is very similar, but some players are better than others. The best players win the trophies, score the most points, and are the best in their area on the court, but the rest of them are not. Why not? What's the reason for this?

Motivation is clearly an essential part of performance—without it, we are never psychologically ready to compete. Motivation operates at many levels and has many influences. People have an underlying level of motivation that influences how they behave across a wide range of situations. A person who is motivated across a wide range of contexts is likely to succeed in many arenas, such sport, business, etc.

Remember, successful people do not give up when they fail. A real champion will feed on failure as motivation to work harder, to focus on getting better results. So always keep in mind the quote "The strongest people are not always the people who win, but the people who don't give up when they lose" (Ashley Hodgeson). Some people want it to happen, some wish it would happen, others **make it happen**. Mentally tough people create timing, moments, good chances, and opportunities. They are aware of what is going on around them.

Take your destiny into your own hands and commit to reaching your destination. You can take charge and shape your own reality. Everything that you can imagine you can have! Really *everything*. Instead of giving reasons why you can't, give yourself reasons why you CAN! YOU CAN DO IT! Believing in yourself is the first step on the road to success.

To find out more about how I can help you or your organization develop mental toughness, visit www.peterestrop.com today, where we offer a range of personal or group coaching programs.

I look forward to working with you and helping you achieve your goals!

To Your Success,

Peter Estrop

Acknowledgments

I'm grateful to so many people for their guidance, inspiration, and help throughout this process, and in my life. I have been positively influenced by so many of them, and I'm grateful for all of the amazing people I have met in my life. Each of them has made me better in so many ways and helped to make me a tougher person.

When writing this book, I was able to delve deeper into the motivation and inspiration behind the toughness I admired around me. I would like to thank Mark Anastasi for his encouragement and support while I was writing this book, and for being consistently available to answer my questions. I appreciate the time Mark spent helping me turning my idea into reality. Mark also participated in virtually every step of the writing, editing, and creative process. Readers of the book will not fully realise Mark's long hours of dedication and commitment, but I know and appreciate the important part he played in bringing this book to life.

Over the years I have been involved in sport, I have met many wonderful people and competitors. I have learned values and principles from people I have played and worked with. I cannot thank Paul and Sarah Christensen enough, who gave me the opportunity to coach teams in South West Basketball for many years. There, I got to work with some fantastic coaches.

Many thanks to all of my colleagues at work who always create an amazing atmosphere. We have shared many great moments over the last ten years.

Growing up in Poland, I met some outstanding people and teachers. They taught me how to win, and how to follow my passion. They encouraged me to fight against adversity and make it through life's obstacles. I would like to thank my amazing parents, Krystyna and Leszek Estrop. In ways they cannot imagine, they have inspired everything good in my life through their belief in me and their unfailing support. I would like to thank my family as well for their support and feedback.

And finally, there is one person who has been with me every step on my journey, my wife Dorota. She made this book better, just as she has always made me better. Her time and contribution are the most important aspects of this book.

References

"Toughness", subtitle Developing True Strength On and Off The Court – Jay Bilas, New American Library – Penguin Group Inc, New York, 2014

"Team psychology in sports", subtitle Theory and Practice – Stewart Cotterill, Routledge, Oxon, 2013

"Mental Toughness", subtitle The Mindset Behind Sporting Achievement, Second Edition– Micheal Sheard, Routledge, Hove, 2013

"Inside Sport Psychology" – Costas I. Karageorghis, Peter C, Terry, Human Kinetics, USA, 2010

Journal of Personality and Social Psychology, 2007, Vol. 92, No. 6, 1087–1101 Copyright 2007 by the American Psychological Association 0022-3514/07/$12.00 DOI: 10.1037/0022-3514.92.6.1087

Effect of Psychological Interventions in Enhancing Mental Toughness Dimensions of Sports Persons E. Bhambri, P.K. Dhillon and S. P Sahni Delhi University, Delhi © Journal of the Indian Academy of Applied Psychology, January - July 2005, Vol. 31, No.1-2, 65-70.

About the author

Peter Estrop is a mental toughness expert, deputy manager, basketball coach, and devoted husband. Born and raised in Gdansk, Poland, during Martial Law, Peter grew up during communist rule when people had to queue for days just to get a loaf of bread. Peter has lived with adversity for most of his life—overcoming a house fire, a serious fall aged 2 that almost killed him, living in a 3x3 meter storage room, and saving his friend from committing suicide.

Since his early years, Peter has always been active in sport. Sport has had a significant impact on his life—first as a player, then as a coach, and now as a mental toughness expert. At various times, he has been a player and coach, an expert and a fan. In his younger days, he spent his time analysing and comparing the mentality of sports and business people. Now, this is both his hobby and his life. As a mental toughness expert, Peter has read many books about the vital role of mental toughness in business and sport. He watches the best players and analyses their decision-making (how they think, what they do or don't do).

He has spent much time talking to true champions, great business leaders such as Dennis Hogan, (Managing Director of Compass Group UK & Ireland) and sports players such as Rafael Nadal, David Beckham, Kobe Bryant, Rudy Fernandez, Andriej Kirilenko, Marat Safin, Guillermo Coria, Gustavo Kuerten, Jimmy Connors, and more. He has also been involved with teams and coaches such as David Blatt (Lebron James' former coach and Cleveland Cavaliers' coach) and Peter Lundgren (Roger Federer's coach).

As an individual, he is committed to developing unstoppable mental toughness. Before writing this book, he climbed the tallest mountain in Poland, met the NBA Commissioner Adam Silver, completed a management academy, and served the Queen of the United Kingdom. While Peter has worked in many jobs, being a mental toughness expert is his favourite job, as he thrives on helping people to build mental toughness as the key to success.

Peter loves people, travelling, and ... coffee. He combines all three in his passion of gaining knowledge about sport by travelling to sports events and business seminars worldwide. Peter's unique knowledge and experience enables him to help others understand what it takes to reach their goals. With Peter's experience and knowledge about mental toughness, he believes he can help many people make their dreams become reality.

He has come a long way to where he is now—from impossible to possible. He knows that obstacles are there for a reason and if his road to become an expert in mental toughness was easy, then it would not last. Every struggle he has faced in his life has shaped him into the person he is today. His aim is to rise by lifting others. Sometimes, people get knocked down lower than they have ever been, but with mental toughness, they can stand back up taller than they ever were. Peter is truly an example of this, and with his passion, he can help you enjoy your life fully.

"I Am a Habit"

by John Di Lemme

I am your constant companion.

I am your greatest helper or your heaviest burden.

I will push you onward or drag you down to failure.

I am completely at your command.

Half the things you do, you might just as well turn over to me, and I will be able to do them quickly and correctly.

I am easily managed; you must merely be firm with me.

Show me exactly how you want something done, and after a few lessons I will do it automatically.

I am the servant of all great men.

And, alas, of all failures as well.

Those who are great, I have made great.

Those who are failures, I have made failures.

I am not a machine, though I work with all the precision of a machine. Plus, the intelligence of a man.

You may run me for profit, or run me for ruin; it makes no difference to me.

Take me, train me, be firm with me and I will put the world at your feet.

Be easy with me, and I will destroy you.

Who am I?

I am a HABIT!

www.ingramcontent.com/pod-product-compliance
Lightning Source LLC
Chambersburg PA
CBHW071000040426
42443CB00007B/587